Y0-BVN-674

Health-Related Fitness
for Grades 5 and 6

GV
443
.H655
1997
West

Chris Hopper, PhD
Humboldt State University

Bruce Fisher
Fortuna Elementary School

Kathy D. Munoz, EdD
Humboldt State University

•A15048 966273

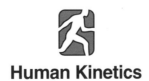

Human Kinetics

We dedicate this book to our families—

Renee, Molly, Ian, and Andrew;

Rich, Heather, Wesley, and Ryan;

Mindi and Jenny.

Library of Congress Cataloging-in-Publication Data

Hopper, Christopher A., 1952–
    Health-related fitness for grades 5 and 6 / Chris Hopper, Bruce
Fisher, Kathy Munoz.
       p.   cm.
    Includes index.
    ISBN 0-88011-480-0
    1. Physical fitness for children.   2. Health education
(Elementary)   3. Cardiovascular system—Diseases—Prevention.
I. Fisher, Bruce, 1949– .   II. Munoz, Kathy, 1951– .
III. Title.
GV443.H655   1997
361.7'042—dc20   96-33878
                                           CIP

ISBN: 0-88011-480-0

Copyright © 1997 by Chris Hopper, Bruce Fisher, and Kathy D. Munoz

All rights reserved. Except for use in a review, the reproduction or utilization of this work in any form or by any electronic, mechanical, or other means, now known or hereafter invented, including xerography, photocopying, and recording, and in any information storage and retrieval system, is forbidden without the written permission of the publisher.

Acquisitions Editor: Scott Wikgren; **Developmental Editor:** Nanette Smith; **Assistant Editor:** Henry Woolsey; **Editorial Assistant:** Coree Schutter; **Copyeditors:** Denelle Eknes, Julia Anderson; **Indexer:** Barbara E. Cohen; **Typesetting and Layout:** Impressions Book and Journal Services, Inc.; **Graphic Designer:** Judy Henderson; **Cover Designer:** Jack Davis; **Illustrators:** Mary Yemma Long, Nicole Barbuto, Craig Ronto, Dianna Porter; **Printer:** Versa Press

Printed in the United States of America

10 9 8 7 6 5 4 3 2 1

Human Kinetics
Web site: http://www.humankinetics.com/

United States: Human Kinetics
P.O. Box 5076, Champaign, IL 61825-5076
1-800-747-4457
e-mail: humank@hkusa.com

Canada: Human Kinetics
Box 24040, Windsor, ON N8Y 4Y9
1-800-465-7301 (in Canada only)
e-mail: humank@hkcanada.com

Europe: Human Kinetics
P.O. Box IW14, Leeds LS16 6TR, United Kingdom
(44) 1132 781708
e-mail: humank@hkeurope.com

Australia: Human Kinetics
57A Price Avenue, Lower Mitcham, South Australia 5062
(08) 277 1555
e-mail: humank@hkaustralia.com

New Zealand: Human Kinetics
P.O. Box 105-231, Auckland 1
(09) 523 3462
e-mail: humank@hknewz.com

Contents

Appendixes   133

Preface

In recent years the following headlines have appeared in the media:

Young Adults More Fat Than Fit, Study Finds

Lorem ipsum dolor sit amet, consectetuer adipiscing elit, euismod tinci magna aliquam enim ad minim erci tation ulla nisl ut aliquip Duis autem ve drerit in vulput sequat, vel illu facilisis at vero

Lorem ipsum dolor sit amet, consectetuer adipiscing elit, sed diam nonummy nibh euismod tincidunt ut laoreet dolore

lore te feugait nulla facilisi. tempor cum soluta nobis ele congue nihil imperdiet dom erat facer possim a m dolor sit amet, elit, sed diam non incidunt ut lao nim ve ullamc uip ex e vel eu lputate vero er

Any Exercise is Good Exercise: Experts say even a little moderate activity goes a long way

Lorem ipsum dolor sit amet, consectetuer adipiscing elit, sed diam nonummy nibh euismod tincidunt ut laoreet dolore magna ali- volutpat. Ut wisi enim ad minim uis nostrud exerci tation ullamcor- it lobortis nisl ut aliquip ex ea consequat. Duis autem vel eum or in hendrerit in vulputate velit

Lorem ipsum dolor sit amet, consectetuer adipiscing elit, sed diam nonummy nibh eu- ismod tincidunt ut laoreet dolore magna ali- quam erat volutpat. Ut wisi enim ad minim veniam, quis nostrud exerci tation ullamcor- per suscipit lobortis nisl ut aliquip ex ea commodo consequat. Duis autem vel eum iriure dolor in hendrerit in vulputate velit

FITNESS: Study Finds Big Slip

Kids Confused On Health, Survey Finds

Lorem ipsum dolor sit amet, consectetuer

facilisis at vero eros et accumsan et iusto

Young People's Health Declining, Report Says

Lorem ipsum dolor sit amet, consectetuer adipiscing elit, sed diam non- ummy nibh euismod tincidunt ut laoreet dolore magna aliquam erat vo- lutpat. Ut wisi enim ad minim veniam, quis nostrud exerci tation ul- lamcorper suscipit lobortis nisl ut aliquip ex ea commodo consequat. Duis autem vel eum iriure dolor in hendrerit in vulputate velit esse mo- lestie consequat, vel illum dolore eu feug accumsan et iusto odio dignissim qui b delenit augue duis dolore te feugait nulla amet, consectetuer adipiscing elit, sed tincidunt ut laoreet dolore magna aliqua ad minim veniam, quis nostrud exerci ta tis nisl ut aliquip ex ea commodo conseq Duis autem vel eum iriure dolor in hend lestie consequat, vel illum dolore eu feug accumsan et iusto odio dignissim qui b delenit augue duis dolore te feugait nulla soluta nobis eleifend option congue ni mazim placerat facer possim assum.

FAT: Even Moderate Weight Gains Are Risky

Lorem ipsum dolor sit amet, consectetuer

amet, consectetuer adipiscing elit, sed n nonummy nibh euismod tincidunt at. Ut wisi enim ad minim veniam, nostrud exerci tation ullamcorper ipit lobortis nisl ut aliquip ex ea com- lo consequat. s autem vel eum iriure dolor in hen- uat, vel illum dolore eu feugiat nulla lisis at vero eros et accumsan et iusto zzril delenit augue duis dolore te feu- nulla facilisi. Nam liber tempor cum

Vigorous Exercise Adds On Years, Study Says

Lorem ipsum dolor sit amet, consectetuer adipiscing elit, sed diam nonummy nibh euismod tincidunt ut laoreet dolore magna aliquam erat volutpat. Ut wisi enim ad minim veniam, quis nostrud ex- erci tation ullamcorper suscipit lobortis nisl ut aliquip ex ea commodo consequat. Duis autem vel eum iriure dolor in hen- drerit in vulputate velit esse molestie con-

sequat, vel illum dolore eu feugiat nulla facilisis at vero eros et accumsan et iusto odio dignissim qui blandit praesent lupta- tum zzril delenit augue duis dolore te feu- gait nulla facilisi. Lorem ipsum dolor sit amet, consectetuer adipiscing elit, sed diam nonummy nibh euismod tincidunt ut laoreet dolore magna aliquam erat vo- lutpat. Ut wisi enim ad minim veniam,

Overall, considerable evidence suggests that the cardiovascular health of children is at risk.

As a teacher, you're as concerned about the cardiovascular health of kids as are parents and medical professionals. You know if kids develop healthy habits when they're in elementary school, chances are they'll become healthy adolescents and adults. With the lively and seasoned activities and lessons in this book, you can incorporate sound cardiovascular wellness into your classroom. Whether you are an elementary school teacher developing physical education lessons or a physical education specialist, you'll find this an invaluable and complete guide to promoting cardiovascular health through daily lessons.

Chris Hopper and Kathy Munoz teach in the Department of Health and Physical Education at Humboldt State University and have worked extensively with teachers in Northern California to improve instruction in physical education and nutrition. Their work has been published in research journals such as *Research Quarterly for Exercise and Sport* and teacher journals such as *Learning*. Bruce Fisher was California Teacher of the Year in 1991 and serves as a consultant for health education to the California Department of Education. Bruce is recognized by his colleagues as an innovative teacher. All three authors have tested the lessons in this book, which represents a decade of professional work.

The authors designed this book to enhance existing physical education programs and to be a comprehensive resource for teachers who want to spice up their teaching with fun-filled, exciting learning activities. This book includes physical education activity lessons that emphasize children enjoying movement.

The fitness and nutrition information includes cardiovascular fitness, strength, endurance, flexibility, fat, carbohydrates, water, sodium, and heart-healthy eating. The goal of the book is to communicate the need for a lifelong commitment to health and physical fitness, using cardiovascular exercise and diet. The goal for you in using the book is to change the attitudes and behaviors of children so they embrace this commitment to health and fitness.

The book emphasizes ready-to-go activities and materials teachers can easily use. The book has a user friendly approach with illustrations, pages to copy, and lesson outlines. We recognize that classroom teachers are extremely busy. The format and design eliminate extra work.

Teachers can meet multiple teaching objectives by using this curriculum. Unique features include cross-curriculum activities, meaningful homework, and cooperative learning activities. In addition, while children are studying fitness and nutrition, they'll be developing research techniques (surveys), critical thinking skills (comparing foods), science concepts (e.g., how the heart works), language arts (e.g., food label analysis), and mathematical applications (e.g., counting pulse rates).

The program covers nine weeks of fitness and nutrition education and activities related to cardiovascular health. Each week includes five 30-minute lessons, with one concept development and discussion lesson, three physical education activity lessons, and one nutrition concept lesson. The lessons are divided into the following sections:

Heart Facts (1 week)

What's in a Workout? (1 week)

Fitness Components (1 week)

Risk Factors (1 week)

Aerobic Fitness concepts (2 weeks)

Flexibility Fitness concepts (1 week)

Strength Fitness concepts (1 week)

Healthy Lifestyle (1 week)

This book is the third in a series of three books designed to enhance the cardiovascular health of children. Be sure to review *Health-Related Fitness for Grades 1 and 2* and *Health-Related Fitness for Grades 3 and 4*.

Acknowledgments

We thank the following teachers for help in pilot testing: Linda Provancha, Fred Johansen, Steve Wartburg, and Linda Buron.

We also thank Tami Jaegel for researching information, and Ira Samuels and Mike Mullane for their advice. We appreciate the inspiration provided by Roland (Lefty) Chell.

We thank Tricia Gill, Elissa Fisher, and Linda Baxter for typing the manuscript.

Introduction to Curriculum

Before starting the curriculum, include an introduction to the lessons and explain the lesson objectives and purposes.

Objectives

1. To teach the basic elements of a healthy cardiovascular system (lungs, heart, and blood vessels)
2. To introduce important fitness and nutrition concepts for a healthy heart
3. To teach children how to plan and develop their own exercise programs

In this introductory lesson, children can develop their own fitness logo and folder (see fig. I.1).

Teaching Strategies

- Before starting the program, give each child a folder to keep all materials from the program. Children create their own fitness logo during the program (see fig. I.2).
- Use laminated task cards with names of specific exercises and activities that you can use as a resource. Use the exercises in chapter 13 to develop cards.
- Stress that children don't have heart attacks. Children develop lifestyle habits that put them at risk for heart disease later in life.
- Avoid simply repeating jumping jacks, windmills, and so forth, with no purpose. Put them into a game or activity.
- Don't use running laps or other exercises as a punishment for bad behavior.
- Use writing projects about exercise and nutrition to improve language arts.
- Avoid elimination activities.

Cross-Curricular Themes

We have identified the following cross-curricular areas in the lessons:

- Health

- Visual and Performing Arts

- Science

- Mathematics

- Social Science

- Language Arts

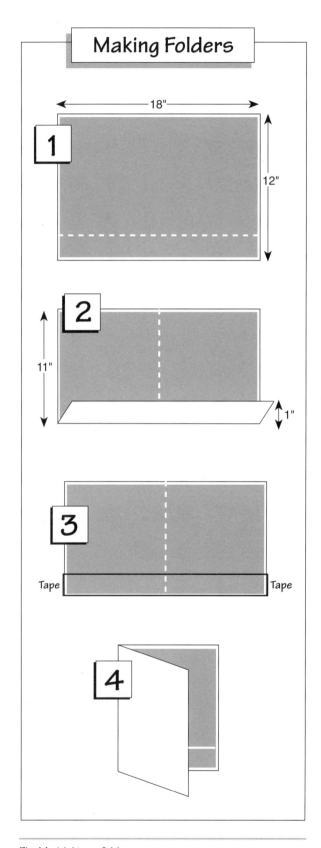

Fig. I.1. Making a folder

Nutrition Education

In nutrition education students gain the knowledge, skills, and motivation they need to make wise food choices. They learn that healthy foods are intimately connected with physical, mental, emotional, and social health. Also, energy, self-image, and physical fitness are related to heart-healthy nutrition. A comprehensive nutrition education program integrates nutrition lessons with the core curriculum. Lessons in this book include classroom activities for food tasting, preparation, and menu planning.

Home Activities

Home activities provide a connection between the home and the school, strengthening the school-family relationship. Parents as care providers can dramatically influence eating habits and physical activity levels. They buy and prepare food for children and determine restaurant choices. In addition, parents help their children make significant choices regarding exercise. Parents can register their children for sport and activity programs and tell their children to turn off the television. In overall lifestyle, parents serve as gatekeepers, and children are unlikely to change their lifestyles without the support of their parents.

A Lesson a Day for Nine Weeks

We organized the curriculum to provide a lesson a day for nine weeks. This concentrated approach will give students the knowledge and skills to make significant lifestyle changes. The curriculum is sequential, with basic knowledge introduced, then applied to cardiovascular health.

Discussion Lessons

Discussion lessons are an essential component of the curriculum and allow students to reflect on important concepts about physical fitness and nutrition. These lessons develop the skills and knowledge of physical fitness and nutrition that are the foundation of a healthy lifestyle.

Assessment Strategies

The purpose of assessment is to evaluate student progress, identify areas of difficulty, and gather

Fitness Logo

Design a fitness logo for the cover of your folder. Your design should incorporate aspects of physical fitness and include the following elements:

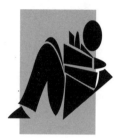

- a geometric shape
- artwork
- interior design
- words or slogans

The following are shapes you may want to consider.

  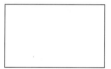 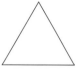

Use your creativity and imagination to create something unique. You may want to design several rough drafts before completing a final copy. (Have someone check your spelling and layout.)

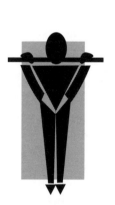 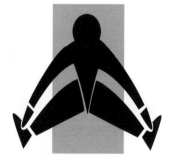 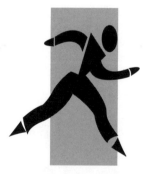

Fig. I.2. Fitness logo

data for instructional planning. The Health-Related Fitness Program uses three types of assessment.

- Performance assessment
  Performance assessment focuses on what students do know. Performance assessment gives students an opportunity to demonstrate their ability to use thinking processes to solve problems related to the subject matter. Performance assessment allows students to work on extended investigations. Students can collect and organize information that they can explain orally, in writing, or with illustrations. Performance assessment may be individual or involve a group of students. The assessment may involve problem solving, observing, interviewing, anecdotal recording, or collecting student work samples.
- Portfolio assessment
  Portfolios of student work, especially when students choose the portfolio pieces, provide an opportunity to holistically assess student understanding and progress. Any product of student work related to the subject matter can be included in a student's portfolio. It may include activity reports, creative writing, teamwork, observations, experiment results, record sheets, home activities, and cooperative group work. An introductory lesson creates folders for individual student portfolios.
- Tests
  You can use a pre- and posttest to determine student mastery of content, facts, and terminology (see Appendix A for a sample). The posttest may include open-ended as well as multiple choice questions.

More Assessment Options

This book provides many opportunities for oral assessment. Many lessons incorporate specific and open-ended questions.

- Cooperative learning
  Many of the lessons are designed for partners or small groups (three or four) of students to work together. These opportunities enhance academic learning and promote interpersonal skills. Research indicates that cooperative learning results in higher achievement and greater motivation. Cooperative groups are useful for accomplishing hands-on activities, researching information, preparing presentations, and reinforcing lesson concepts. Suggestions for cooperative learning opportunities appear throughout the program.
- Open-ended questions
  A student is given a situation and asked to communicate a response. Open-ended questions allow for a variety of acceptable responses and can detect possible misconceptions. Student thinking can be reflected in the organization and interpretation of essential concepts, information, generalizations, and appropriate language.
- Cross-curricular integration
  Cross-curricular activities are incorporated into many of the lessons. They are indicated by icons (graphic symbols). These interdisciplinary connections enhance students' conceptual development and develop an understanding of physical education as an integrated part of educating the whole child. Due to the time constraints placed on self-contained classroom teachers, we left selection of activities to the discretion of the educator.

Warming Up and Cooling Down

Each lesson should start with a warm-up and finish with a cool-down.

Warm-Up = Light Activity + Stretching

A warm-up before exercise prepares your body for activity and avoids "jump starting" the body. Warm-ups stretch muscles and help prevent muscle soreness and injury. In addition, warm-ups prepare the heart for more vigorous activity and avoid adding stress.

Exercise specialists recommend completing light activity first, such as jogging, followed by gentle static stretching (see chapters 11 and 12). Remember not to bounce when stretching.

Although children rarely stretch before going out to recess or playing vigorous activities, stretching is an investment for the future. Joints that are flexible in childhood will gradually lose mobility with age, leading to a reduced range of movement. Developing a lifetime habit of stretching before exercise can pay dividends now and later. Refer to lesson 31 for more detailed information on preferred stretching techniques.

Cool-Down = Less Vigorous Activity + Stretching

The cool-down is an essential part of any exercise session. It is just as important as the warm-up. A cool-down should last about five minutes and allow your body to gently recover after vigorous exercise. An abrupt end to exercise sends your blood pressure fluctuating like a yo-yo. This leads to slow removal of waste products. Light activity and stretching continue the pumping action of muscles on veins, helping the circulation remove wastes. Static stretching may help reduce delayed soreness or muscle pain the day after exercise.

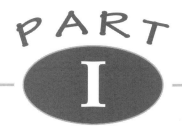

Weekly Lessons

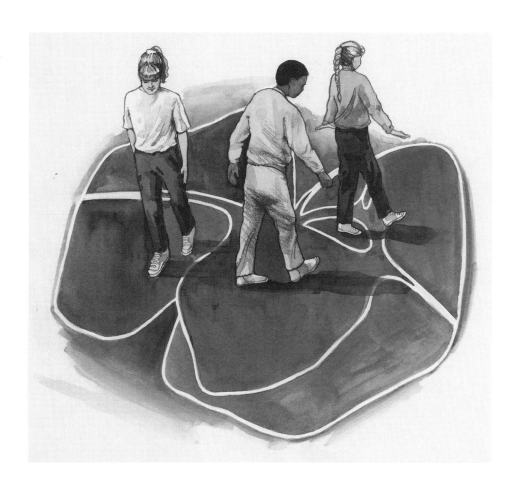

CHAPTER 1

Week 1: Heart Facts

The lessons introduce students to the structure and function of the heart. The physical activity lessons emphasize specific facts associated with blood circulation in the body. The nutrition lesson helps students identify foods that promote cardiovascular health.

Lesson 1

Heart Facts

Goals

- To introduce the heart structure and function
- To draw and map the circulatory system

Key Concepts

The heart is a pump consisting of four chambers. Blood carrying oxygen is pumped from the heart to the body, and blood returning from body parts carries carbon dioxide.

1. Size and appearance of heart
   Although no larger than a human fist, the human heart is probably the most important muscle in your body. Somewhat pear shaped, the heart has four "rooms" or chambers and weighs about as much as a softball (show softball).
2. Purpose and function of heart
   Your heart has a job that never stops. It must squeeze about 10 pints (show pint or liter container) of blood through your body every day. It beats about 80 or 90 times a minute to accomplish this. That's roughly 5,000 times an hour, 120,000 times a day, or over 43 million times a year!
3. Brief overview of circulatory system
   As the fuel pump of your body, your heart is the power source behind the blood flow throughout your entire body. This movement of blood takes place through tubes called arteries and veins. The circulatory process provides nourishment and removes waste products from the cells.
4. Your heart is the strongest muscle in your body. It pumps blood to all parts of your body. After blood has traveled through your body, it comes back to your heart. It is blue because oxygen has been removed. Your heart pumps the used blood to the lungs where it receives oxygen. When blood comes back from the lungs, it is bright red. Then your heart pumps blood to your body. Your hard-working heart has to pump blood to your brain cells and millions of other cells in your body night and day for your whole life—without a break.

5. Your heart consists of four chambers. The top two chambers are known as right and left auricles. The bottom two chambers are called the right and left ventricles.
6. Blood returning from the body carries carbon dioxide, which the body does not need. Blood from the head or arms enters the right auricle through the superior vena cava. Blood from the rest of the body comes back to the right auricle from the inferior vena cava.
7. Blood inside the heart passes to the right ventricle through the tricuspid valve. This blue blood is pumped to the lungs through the pulmonary artery to remove carbon dioxide. At the lungs, blood with a fresh supply of oxygen returns to the heart.
8. Oxygenated (with oxygen) blood returns to the left atrium and passes through the mitral valve to the left ventricle. It is then pumped to the head, arms, trunk, and legs.

Materials

1. Model or large picture of heart
2. Pint or liter container
3. Ten-inch or standard softball
4. Bicycle or hand pump
5. Fig. 1.1 of body (one per student)
6. Fig. 1.2 of circulatory system (one per student)
7. Fig. 1.3 of a child's heart
8. Fig. 1.4 of blood flow through the heart, lungs, and body
9. Red and blue crayons
10. Handout 1.1 Week 1, Family Activity: Family Fitness Survey (one per student)

Activity: Heart Facts

- Introduce topic with student activity designed to clarify location, size, and shape of heart.
- Pass out Fig. 1.1.
- Ask students to draw on the outline (fig. 1.1) what they think their heart looks like, and draw it on the outline where they think it's

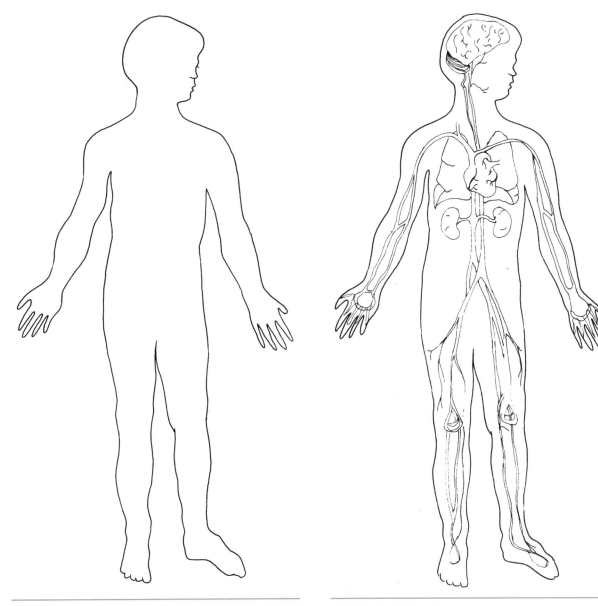

Fig. 1.1. Body outline

Fig. 1.2. The child circulatory system

located (encourage them to be accurate and include as much detail as possible).

- Draw an accurate heart (discussing the heart's features). Use a model or a large picture of a heart.
- Students draw a second model, as accurately as possible. This time they should attempt to draw the heart to relative scale.
- Present information on function of the heart.
- Demonstrate activity of a pump using a bicycle or hand pump. Explain that the pump action is similar to the pumping action of the heart.

- Have students open and close fist for three minutes. Ask students the following questions that lead to a discussion:

  a. Is your hand tired? The heart works harder than the hand because it continues pumping blood.

  b. Why doesn't your heart get tired and stop beating? The heart has a special kind of muscle (smooth) and larger amounts of blood.

  c. What are some other strong muscles in your body? The leg and abdomen muscles.

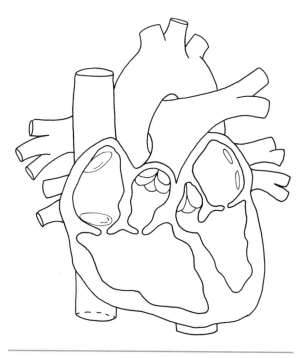

Fig. 1.3. *A child's heart*

d. Do they work continuously? The leg and
   abdomen muscles are able to rest.
• Discuss circulatory system.
• Have students use a red crayon to trace the
  pathway of blood from the heart to all parts
  of the body (use fig. 1.2).
• Use a blue crayon to draw a second line back
  to the heart.
• Using fig. 1.3, help students trace the flow of
  blue and red blood through the heart. Ask
  children to use blue and red crayons to identify the color of blood on each side of the
  heart.
• Using fig. 1.4, help students trace the flow of
  blood from the heart to the lungs, and from
  the lungs to the heart, and back to the body.
• Send home handout 1.1 Family Fitness Survey.

Teaching Tips

Press down on a finger for a few seconds. Have
children notice the change in the color of the fin-

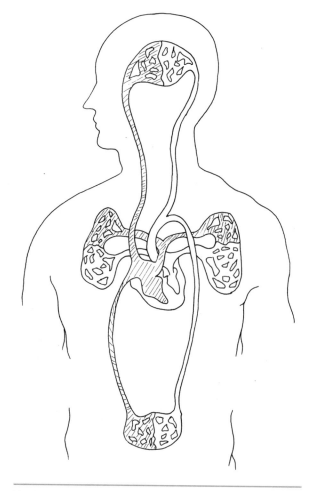

Fig. 1.4. *Blood flow*

ger. What is happening in the finger? Part of the
finger turns white because it is not able to receive
blood due to the pressure. What is the importance
of blood flow?

Other Resources

*American Heart Association Upper Elementary School
Site Program: Getting to Know Your Heart*, 1988, Dallas: American Heart Association.

Handout 1.1   Week 1, Family Activity; Fitness Survey

Parents: complete the following survey as individuals. Then your child can also answer the questions.

	Always	Usually	Sometimes	Never
1. I walk or use a bicycle rather than go by car when it is safe and possible.	3	2	1	0
2. I make time to exercise at least 3 times a week ouside of school or work.	3	2	1	0
3. After school or work, I am physically active instead of watching T.V. and playing video games.	3	2	1	0
4. I regularly participate in sports and rec-reation.	3	2	1	0
5. I know approximately how much fat is in the foods I eat.	3	2	1	0
6. I read labels to check the nutritional value on the foods our family buys.	3	2	1	0
7. I eat fruits and vegetables every day.	3	2	1	0
8. I avoid foods that are deep fried.	3	2	1	0
9. I participate in one physical activity a week, e.g. walking.	3	2	1	0
10. I limit the number of junkfood snacks (potato chips, cookies, candy, soda) between meals.	3	2	1	0

Time: 20 minutes

Please return by _____

Teacher Notes:

Use the survey and discuss responses with the class. At this stage it is important to create awareness of habits, rather than saying some are better than others. Also, ask children to name other health habits not addressed in survey that affect health.

Use the survey to identify one area for each student that can be improved. Start a goal setting procedure and help each student to make lifestyle changes.

Example: Need to reduce the amount of deep fried foods.

Strategies:

- Pass on the french fries and try a small salad at fast food restaurants.
- Eat grilled or barbecued food instead of deep fried food.
- Eat a regular hamburger rather than a double deluxe bacon cheeseburger.

Scoring:

25–30	Living a healthy life	<14	Major changes necessary for good health habits
20–24	Doing fine, but could improve		
15–19	Need to make significant adjustments		

Lesson 2

Take It to Heart

Goals

- To demonstrate that blood cells carry oxygen
- To improve cardiovascular endurance

Key Concepts

Cells in the blood absorb oxygen at the lungs. This oxygenated blood then returns to the heart before being pumped to all body parts. Blood leaves the heart in a vessel called the aorta and transports oxygen to the body.

Materials

1. Five hula hoops
2. Bean bags or balls (one per child)

Warm-Up: 5 Minutes

Select stretching and warm-up activities.

Activity: Take It to Heart

- Arrange hula hoops at equal distances from each other in a playing area the size of a basketball court.

- Groups of four students select a hoop as home base and stand around it.
- Place same number of bean bags as team members in each hoop.
- On command to start the game, players (who represent blood cells) try to steal a bean bag (molecule of oxygen) from another hoop.
- Each player may carry only one bean bag at a time and must place it in the center of his or her home base (hoop) before trying to get another.
- After two minutes, a signal ends the round and teams tally their bean bag totals.

Cool-Down: 5 Minutes

Select stretching and cool-down activities.

Teaching Tips

Emphasize that players may only carry one bag at a time and cannot pick up a bean bag after the ending signal. No guarding of home base.

Lesson 3

Side by Side

Goals

- To reinforce that one side of the heart has red blood and the other side has blue blood
- To practice cooperative play

Key Concepts

The heart has a right side and a left side. The right side receives blue blood (without oxygen) from the body and pumps it to the lungs. The left side

receives red blood (with oxygen) from the lungs and pumps it to the body.

Materials

1. Fifteen blue and 15 red flags
2. Ten cones

Warm-Up: 5 Minutes

Select stretching and warm-up activities.

Activity: Side by Side

- Give each student either a blue or red flag.
- Students pair up side to side within an area the size of a basketball court (marked by cones), representing two sides of a heart.
- On the command "Body" the pairs split up and jog.
- Students find a new partner on the command "Heart."
- The partners complete an exercise while side by side.
- Any student without a partner keeps running. Students can only pair up with a student holding the opposite color.
- Select exercises from chapter 13, for example, jumping jacks, mountain climbers, or cross-country skiers.

Cool-Down: 5 Minutes

Select stretching and cool-down activities.

Teaching Tips

When partners split, they can use different movement patterns, such as gallop, skip, jogging backward, hopping, or sideways shuffle. In addition to pairing up, students can make groups of four, with two red and two blue flags. Students then represent the four chambers of the heart. Designate half the students as auricles and the other half as ventricles. Each group should consist of two auricles and two ventricles. Before "Body" command, name the exercise to do for that round.

Lesson 4
Chamber Challenge
WEEK 1

Goals

- To simulate blood flow patterns
- To improve cardiovascular endurance (with paced running)

Key Concepts

Successful runners develop a movement style that results in smooth, sustained running ability. An opportunity to practice efficient running that reinforces blood flow patterns is included in this activity.

Materials

1. Forty cones or markers
2. Labels for body parts

Warm-Up: 5 Minutes

Select stretching and warm-up activities.

Activity: Chamber Challenge

- Mark out with cones an area that represents the four chambers of the heart, lungs, head, feet, and arms (see fig. 1.5).
- Have students form pairs and jog side by side, following the flow of blood from heart to lungs, and through the body. A sample path is shown in figure 1.5.
- Label the entry and exit areas of the heart.
- Instruct them to run so their left and right feet move in rhythm together. When they can do this in pairs, have them progress to groups of four. Encourage students to use efficient running techniques.
- Call out a specific activity, such as sleeping, eating, playing tennis or soccer, walking. Students should move faster with more intense activities because the heart pumps more blood at a faster rate when the body is active.

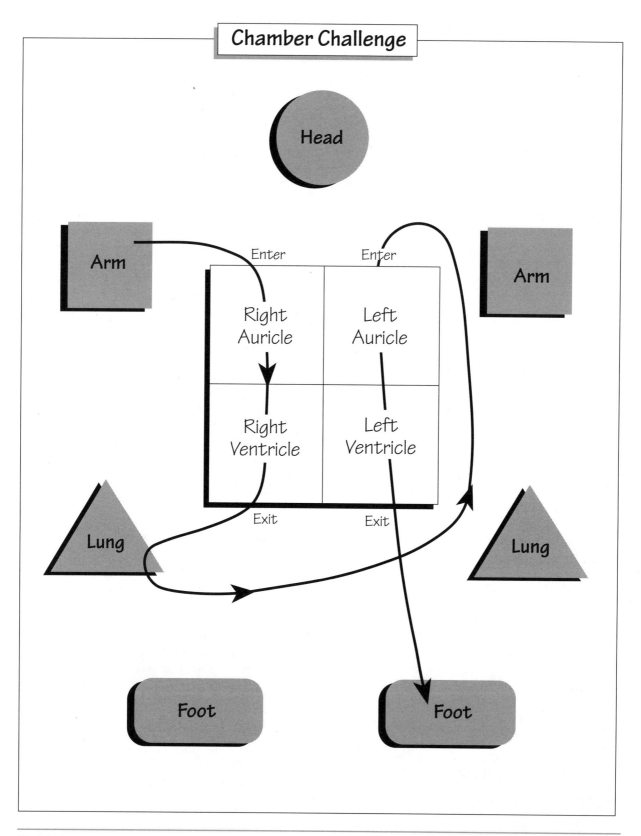

Fig. 1.5. Chamber challenge

Cool-Down: 5 Minutes

Select stretching and cool-down activities.

Teaching Tips

Encourage the following for an efficient running style:

1. Move arms in opposition to legs, bend elbows.
2. Hold head steady with only a slight body lean.
3. Land heel first and push off with ball of foot.
4. Swing legs and feet and land straight ahead.
5. Stride longer than when walking.
6. Bend elbows (90 degrees) with hands relaxed.

WEEK 1

Lesson 5

Food Components

Goal

- To be able to identify and list the attributes that distinguish foods

Key Concepts

Use the concept attainment teaching model to give students practice in inductive reasoning and an awareness of foods containing different attributes, namely fat and cholesterol. Exemplars are a subset of a collection of data. By comparing positive exemplars with negative exemplars, students will learn the concept that foods contain different components that they can classify. Attributes are features that all foods possess or have in common. A hypothesis is an educated guess or predicted result based on prior knowledge or experience.

Materials

1. Examples of menus or recipes for each group or cards with foods already listed
2. One yard of string or yarn for each group
3. Blank three-by-five cards (eight–10 per group)

Activity: Food Components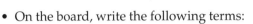

- On the board, write the following terms:

Positive exemplars   Negative exemplars

Carrots   Eggs

Then ask the students the following: "Look at these two words. How are they alike and how are they different? Carrots have the attributes of our category. Eggs do

not." (Be sure to accept and acknowledge all reasonable responses.)
- Then write the following:

Rice   Butter

Say, "Now examine this pair. Rice has the attributes we are concerned with. Butter does not. What do carrots and rice have in common that eggs and butter do not?"
- Ask the students to work independently during this phase of the activity. Present two more words (positive exemplars are foods that contain no fat or cholesterol and negative exemplars contain fat and cholesterol). Ask students to compare and contrast them, trying to discover what the positive exemplars have in common that they do not share with negative exemplars.

Oatmeal   Sour cream

"Now what do you see? Please write down your hypothesis. What do you think are the attributes that the positive words have in common that they do not share with the words I have identified as negative?"
- After a few seconds write the following:

Bananas   Avocados

"Did any of you have to change your ideas?" Then write the following and ask again, "Did any of you have to change your ideas?"

Broccoli	Cheddar cheese
Cheerios	Margarine
Corn	Hamburger
French bread	Pork chops
Apples	Whole milk

- Then say, "Oranges. Based on your hypothesis, is this positive or negative?" Continue providing one word exemplars and asking them to identify if they are positive or negative. If they can identify them correctly, ask them to share their hypotheses. Confirm their hypotheses and relate the essential attributes of the positive exemplars. Ask the students to come up with a few of their own positive and negative exemplars.
- Ask the students to describe their thoughts about the processes they just used. Discuss the role of hypotheses and how many different hypotheses the class came up with.
- Assign groups for this next activity. Give each group a string to use to form a circle, blank three-by-five cards, and school lunch menus or samples of recipes from cookbooks. Ask them to look for positive and negative exemplars and write them on the cards. Then place the cards inside the "at-tribute circle" or string if they are positive (do not contain fat or cholesterol) or outside the circle if they are negative exemplars.
- Discuss their findings with the class.

Teaching Tips

Circulate a sign-up sheet for students to bring a variety of foods for the next nutrition lesson. Examples should include the following:

- Fresh fruit, such as bananas, apples, and oranges
- Vegetables, such as broccoli and avocado
- Protein such as beef, peanut butter, and hot dogs
- Dairy foods, such as cottage cheese and regular cheese
- Snack foods, such as potato chips, soda, pretzels, donuts, mustard, mayonnaise, catsup, and jelly

Week 2: What's in a Workout?

The lessons cover the rationale for physical fitness and how to organize an effective exercise program. The activity lessons emphasize different strategies to achieve physical fitness. The nutrition information introduces the concept of reducing fat in the diet.

Lesson 6

What's in a Workout?

Goals

- To understand the three parts of an aerobic workout
- To create a sample workout

Key Concepts

Successful and safe workouts involve warm-up, peak activity, and cool-down segments.

Physical fitness has value in our lives for the following reasons:

1. Emergencies—running to get help when a friend has been hurt
2. Demands of everyday life—lifting and moving objects, changing a car tire
3. Playing sports and enjoying recreational activities
4. Maintaining health—reducing the risk of heart disease

Explain that developing and maintaining physical fitness is best achieved with exercise programs. Explain that an exercise program has three phases:

1. Warm-up (5 minutes)
   Warm-up refers to a gradual increase in physical activity. The purpose of warming up is to prevent muscle strain, soreness, and to increase the elasticity (stretchiness) of muscles.
2. Peak workout (15–20 minutes)
   This cardiovascular part of the workout is the most important because it strengthens the heart and increases the efficiency of the circulation system. Many types of continuous or rhythmic exercises are used in this phase of the workout. The key is that exercise is continuous and regular.
3. Cool-down (5 minutes)
   The cool-down is similar to the warm-up. The cool-down is a gradual transition from strenuous to reduced activity. This helps prevent muscle soreness and tension.

Materials

1. Sample workout, handout 2.1 My Personal Workout (sample)
2. Student record sheet, handout 2.2 My Personal Workout

3. Sports-related magazines (*Running World, Sports Illustrated*)
4. Scissors

Activity: What's in a Workout?

 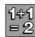

- Brainstorm ideas for a peak workout.
- Review the sample workout in handout 2.1 with a partner. Pairs create their own workout that models all three components (warm-up, peak, and cool-down).
- Using sports-related magazines, cut out one picture that represents each of the three components.
- Share these with another set of partners, then complete handout 2.2 My Personal Workout and modify according to any recommendations.
- Ask for volunteers to share their workouts with the class.

Teaching Tips

Select three or four appropriate workouts to use as part of your physical education lessons. Students can act as "teachers" leading the class through their workout. Save this lesson to use again in the Fitness Club (lesson 43). In a triathlon athletes usually complete three fitness activities, such as running, swimming, and biking. A similar Olympic event is the decathlon (10 events). Create a workout or "athlon" using the following geometric shapes: triangle (three); rectangle (four); pentagon (five); hexagon (six); octagon (eight).

Workouts can be designed for the whole class to complete in a physical education lesson or with friends and family in the neighborhood. For example, the following is a neighborhood family pentathlon: walk 1 mile to park, run or jog 2 laps of the park, do 15 sit-ups, play catch for 5 minutes, and walk home. Create a name for each of the workouts. Research information concerning history of the modern and ancient Olympic games. The address of the US Olympic Foundation: U.S. Olympic Committee, Department of Education, 1750 E. Boulder Street, Colorado Springs, CO 80909-5760.

Handout 2.1   My Personal Workout (sample)

This is a sample workout for at home on weekends.

Warm-up

Stretch the legs and back

Jog around yard

Stretch upper body

Shoot a few hoops

Peak

Ride bike for five minutes to park

Jog four laps of the track

Ride bike for five minutes back home

Cool-down

Walk around yard

Stretch upper and lower body

Handout 2.2   My Personal Workout

Name_____

Develop a plan for a personal workout at home on weekends or during school physical education. Label the amount of time for each phase.

Warm-up _____minutes

Peak _____minutes

Cool-down _____minutes

WEEK 2

Lesson 7

Station to Station

Goal

- To improve cardiovascular endurance

Key Concepts

Cardiovascular exercise stations are an effective way of providing continuous activity and organizing a large group for exercise. Student motivation increases through variety of exercise choices.

Materials

1. Station cards (see teaching tips)
2. Five jump ropes
3. Ten cones
4. Mats
5. Four or five basketballs

Warm-Up: 5 Minutes

Select stretching and warm-up activities.

Activity: Station to Station

- Arrange seven station activities.
- Divide class into groups with three or four students per group, one group per station.
- The first time these stations are introduced, demonstrate each activity.
- Allow one minute per station initially, and gradually increase the duration as the class endurance level improves.
- Start with familiar cardiovascular activities such as the following:

Jump ropes

Specify several basic jumps. Those who can't jump rope can hold rope with both handles in one hand and do side to side swings or place rope on the floor and jump over and back.

Sit-ups or push-ups

See chapter 13.

Basketball dribble and shoot

All students in group dribble 20 yards (minimum), shoot, and return to starting position. If no basketball hoop is available, dribble to a wall, bounce ball against wall, dribble back, repeat.

Agility run

Position 10 playground cones three feet apart in a straight line or pattern. Students weave through cones one at a time. When all students reach one end, they take turns weaving in and out back to the start.

Mountain climbers or cross-country skiers

See chapter 13.

Perimeter run

Students jog the perimeter of the activity area, being careful not to interfere with other stations.

Refuel break

Students can refuel when at this station. It is important for students to replenish water.

Cool-Down: 5 Minutes

Select stretching and cool-down activities.

Teaching Tips

Large, laminated number cards help direct rotations between stations. When the entire activity is completed, the last group at each station is responsible for putting equipment away. If activity stations are located outdoors, mats should be provided for push-ups and sit-ups.

WEEK 2

Lesson 8

Challenge Course

Goals

- To improve cardiovascular endurance
- To rate personal activity levels with an exertion scale
- To review taking a pulse rate

Key Concepts

The *perceived exertion scale* is used to help students determine their levels of effort in an activity. Although it is not precise, it provides a reference point for the intensity of a workout.

Materials

1. Handout 2.3 Perceived Exertion Scale
2. Ten cones
3. Mats
4. Benches (turn upside down)
5. Four to six hoops
6. Six jump ropes
7. Yardstick (for bar)
8. Handout 2.4 Perceived Exertion Scale Ratings

Warm-Up: 5 Minutes

Select stretching and warm-up activities.

Activity: Challenge Course

- Review pulse taking from Lesson 21 (see pages 54–55).
- Set up a miniature challenge course in the gym or outdoors. The course is a series of obstacles in a circle (see fig. 2.1).

- Students rate their perceived exertion (PE) level. Periodically in this activity have students stop and take pulse rates and compare to PE Scale.
- Divide the class into pairs with one student on the course and the other jogging or walking around the outside.
- Students on the circuit move as fast as they can around the course. Demonstrate the specified movements from start to finish. Movement is continuous.
- Organize the course so it is wide enough to accommodate two or three children at a time without blockages.
- The course can include all types of locomotor movements (running, jumping, hopping) and moving under, over, and through obstacles.
- After two minutes partners change roles.

Cool-Down: 5 Minutes

Select stretching and cool-down activities.

Teaching Tips

The PE Scale is based on perceived exertion (how hard you are working out). Display the PE Scale on a chart in large letters on the wall for reference. For the next week students can identify activities (recess, physical education lessons, playing at home, and others) and complete a Perceived Exertion Scale Rating (see handout 2.4).

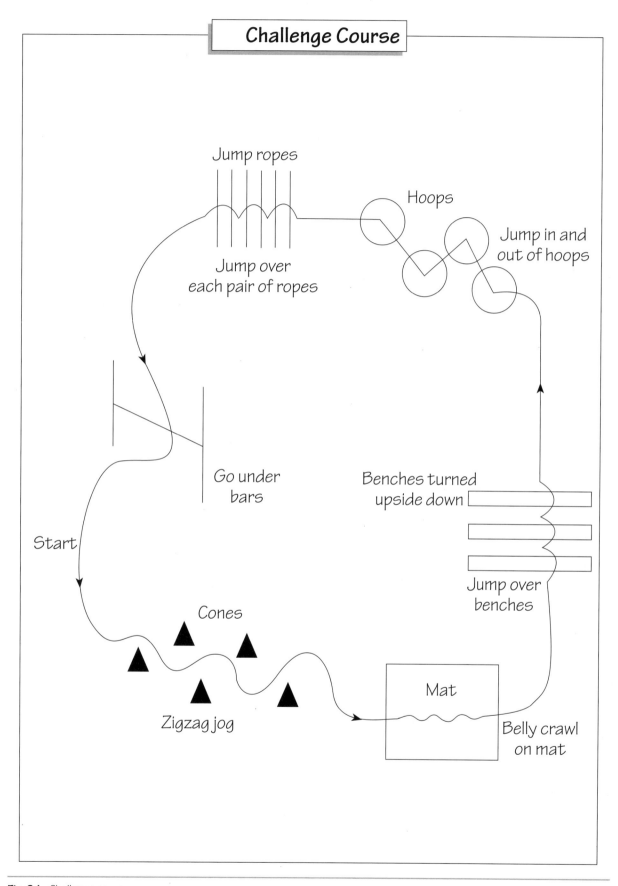

Fig. 2.1. Challenge course

Handout 2.3   Perceived Exertion Scale

1   Very, very light

2   Very light

3   Fairly light

4   Somewhat hard

5   Hard

6   Very hard

7   Very, very hard

Handout 2.4   Perceived Exertion Scale Ratings

Name_____

1. Activity:

   Date:

   PE scale rating:

2. Activity:

   Date:

   PE scale rating:

3. Activity:

   Date:

   PE scale rating:

4. Activity:

   Date:

   PE scale rating:

WEEK 2

Lesson 9

Sport Jamboree

Goals

- To develop cardiovascular endurance
- To improve specific sports skills

Key Concepts

Workouts are possible through sport activities without having to rely on traditional game formats. Participation in "microsport" activities enhances skill development.

Materials

1. Whistle
2. Six to eight basketballs or eight-inch rubber balls
3. Six soccer balls
4. Four cones

Warm-Up: 5 Minutes

Select stretching and warm-up activities.

Activity: Sport Jamboree

- Number students one to five as they line up around a basketball court or an area 40 × 30 yards.
- Tell students to jog around the court.
- Explain that when you blow the whistle, you will call out a number and specify an activity. For example, call out, "Fives and basketball." Students with that number run into the court and complete one of the following: dribble a basketball down the court and score as many baskets as possible.

- The remainder of class keeps moving in different ways, such as jogging, galloping, and skipping.
- After 30 seconds of the sport skill, the students move back to the outside. Then call another number.

Cool-Down: 5 Minutes

Select stretching and cool-down activities.

Teaching Tips

If students wish to pass others, they may do so on the *outside* of moving students. Periodically call "slow walk" (or "water break") to avoid extreme fatigue. For a variation call out two numbers at a time and specify different activities for each number. Keep a checklist to track the numbers that you call out.

Examples of basketball activities:

- Dribble and shoot at one end, and dribble to other end and shoot.
- Stand on the free throw line and shoot.
- Set up two cones and dribble back and forth as quickly as possible.

Examples of soccer activities:

- Pass a soccer ball with a partner (move up and down the court with the ball).
- Dribble a ball on lines on the court or playground.
- Toss ball in the air, receive, control, and dribble.
- Dribble around four cones in the middle of the court.

WEEK 2

Lesson 10

Where's the Fat?

Goals

- To investigate the hidden fat content of common foods
- To identify common properties of sample foods and categorize them into food groups
- To record, compare, and interpret data

Key Concepts

This lesson continues the discussion from lesson 5 on food attributes. In this lesson, students will examine and organize foods into categories, collect information about which foods contain fat, and draw conclusions from their results. Generally, fruits, vegetables, breads, and cereals have very little fat. Dairy foods and meat can be good sources of fat, depending on the choices made within the group. For example, nonfat milk has less than one gram of fat, whereas whole milk has five grams of fat per eight-ounce serving.

Materials

1. Samples of beverages and foods from different food groups, cut into one-inch pieces or small samples. Examples include milk, soda, bananas, apples, broccoli, peanut butter, butter, mustard, mayonnaise, potato chips, pretzels, bread, cheese, doughnuts, jelly, catsup, and hot dogs.
2. Brown grocery bags cut into sheets, approximately 12 × 15 inches (one per group)
3. Eye droppers for liquids (one per liquid)
4. Handout 2.5 Where's the Fat? (one per group)
5. Plastic wrap
6. Metal spoon
7. Overhead transparency and transparency pen (one per group)
8. Handout 2.6 Week 2, Family Activity: Out With the Fat, In With the Lean (one per student)

Activity: Where's the Fat?

- Before the lesson, have the various foods on a table for the class to view. While working in cooperative groups of two or three, ask the students to list the foods on an overhead transparency and group them. Next, ask them to label or categorize their groupings.
- One student from each group will share their ideas with the class, displaying their overhead transparencies. What foods belongs to what group? Do any of the categories relate to each other (some may have fat and others may not).
- How might we test the fat content of food? Ask the students to hypothesize what they think would happen if you were to take one of the foods and rub it on a piece of brown paper. They should respond that food with fat would leave an oily spot. With a small amount of butter on a spoon, demonstrate how to rub the piece of brown paper with the test food and describe what happens to the paper.
- Ask the students to predict which foods from their list will contain fat and record it on their handout.
- Provide each group with a piece of brown paper. Instruct them to fold the brown paper in half four times to produce 16 blocks. Label each block with the name of the test food.
- Each group will test the food samples by rubbing a small amount of the food in the labeled square. If the sample is soft like mustard, rub it with a spoon. If it is hard like a nut or cracker, place a small piece of plastic wrap over the sample and smash it with a spoon. Scrape off any excess sample that sticks to the paper. If liquids are used, place one or two drops on the paper using the eye dropper.
- Let the paper dry and hold it up to the light. If the food contains fat it will leave a greasy mark.
- Record the results on the handout and compare to predictions.
- Ask the groups to rank which foods appeared to be higher in fat than the others.
- Write a summary statement or paragraph about the results of the lesson. Ask them to apply their knowledge to everyday situations.

Teaching Tips

You can extend the lesson by asking the students to plan a meal that would be high or low in fat.

This lesson requires two activity periods. Schedule time for food samples to dry.

Handout 2.5   Where's the Fat?

Food sample	Food group	Prediction (Y/N)	Results (Y/N)
_____	_____	_____	_____
_____	_____	_____	_____
_____	_____	_____	_____
_____	_____	_____	_____
_____	_____	_____	_____
_____	_____	_____	_____
_____	_____	_____	_____
_____	_____	_____	_____
_____	_____	_____	_____
_____	_____	_____	_____
_____	_____	_____	_____
_____	_____	_____	_____

Write a concluding statement or summary:

Handout 2.6   Week 2, Family Activity: Out With the Fat, In With the Lean

Fifteen Tips to Help You Avoid Too Much Fat

1. Steam, boil, or bake vegetables; or for a change, stir-fry in a small amount of vegetable oil.
2. Season vegetables with herbs and spices rather than with sauces, butter, or margarine.
3. Try lemon juice on salads or use limited amounts of oil-based salad dressing.
4. To reduce saturated fat, use margarine instead of butter in baked products, and when possible, use oil instead of shortening.
5. Try whole-grain flours to enhance flavors of baked goods made with fewer fat- and cholesterol-containing ingredients.
6. Replace whole milk with skim or low-fat milk in puddings, soups, and baked products.
7. Substitute plain low-fat yogurt, blender-whipped low-fat cottage cheese, or buttermilk in recipes that call for sour cream or mayonnaise.
8. Choose lean cuts of meat.
9. Trim fat from meat before or after cooking.
10. Roast, bake, broil, or simmer meat, poultry, or fish.
11. Remove skin from poultry before cooking.
12. Cook meat or poultry on a rack so the fat will drain off. Use a nonstick pan for cooking so added fat will be unnecessary.
13. Chill meat or poultry broth until the fat becomes solid. Spoon off the fat before using the broth.
14. Limit egg yolks to one per serving when making scrambled eggs. Use additional egg whites for larger servings.
15. Try substituting egg whites in recipes calling for whole eggs. For example, use two egg whites in place of each whole egg in muffins, cookies, and puddings.

Activity

In discussion with your family choose one of the listed tips that you can accomplish at a meal. Design a short survey that family members can respond to. Use the following two questions as examples and design a couple more questions.

	Strongly agree	Agree	Neutral	Disagree	Strongly disagree
1. The meal tasted as good as the old method.	_____	_____	_____	_____	_____
2. I would prefer to use the new method of cooking in the future.	_____	_____	_____	_____	_____
3.	_____	_____	_____	_____	_____
4.	_____	_____	_____	_____	_____
5.	_____	_____	_____	_____	_____

Time: 30 to 45 minutes

Please return by _____.

Week 3: Fitness Components

The lessons make distinctions between skill fitness and health fitness. Although both types of fitness are important for an active lifestyle, this book emphasizes health fitness as a way of preventing the onset of cardio-vascular disease.

WEEK 3

Lesson 11

Skill Fitness

Goals

- To introduce the benefits of physical fitness
- To reinforce the various components of skill fitness

Key Concepts

There are two current definitions of physical fitness: skill-related and health-related physical fitness. Skill-related fitness enables children to perform effectively in sports. Health-related fitness prevents disease and promotes lifelong health.

Types of physical fitness include the following:

a. Skill-related fitness is needed to perform sport activities successfully (athletes have high levels of skill fitness). Components of skill-related fitness are agility, balance, coordination, power, reaction time, and speed. Ability in these areas is partly determined by natural or inherited traits. Some children are naturally better at sports than others.

b. Health-related fitness helps prevent disease and promotes good health. Components of health-related fitness correspond to lifetime health and are flexibility, cardiovascular endurance, strength, and body composition. These components can be improved by training and practice. Health-related fitness is developed in lesson 12.

Materials

1. Handout 3.1 Skill Fitness Score Sheet
2. Stopwatch
3. Chalk
4. Five chairs
5. Pieces of $8\frac{1}{2} \times 11$ paper (one per pair)
6. Two cones
7. Tennis balls
8. Yardstick
9. Chart paper

Warm-Up: 5 Minutes

Select stretching and warm-up activities.

Activity: Skill Fitness

Have students complete each of the following activities, or use the activities as demonstrations with one or two students performing the activity. Record results on the score sheet (see handout 3.1).

1. **Stork stand** (balance)
   Stand on the dominant (preferred) leg. Place the other foot against the shin of the dominant leg. Place hands on hips. Raise the heel of the dominant foot and maintain balance without the heel touching the floor, moving the other foot, or releasing hands from the hips. Record the number of seconds the balance is held. The heel must stay off the ground.

2. **Blast off** (power)
   Standing by a wall, children jump and reach as high as possible. Hold a piece of chalk so its end is even with your fingertips. Stand with both feet on the floor and your side to the wall, and reach and mark as high as possible. Jump upward with both feet, swing arms upward, and make another chalk mark on the wall. With a yardstick measure the distance between reaching height and jumping height.

3. **Chair slalom** (agility)
   Arrange five chairs, four yards apart. Starting by the first chair, weave in and out, turn, weave in and out on the way back. Then go around the starting chair and complete the course again. The score is the number of seconds for two circuits.

4. **Gravity grab** (reaction time)
   Have a partner hold a sheet of paper so the side edge is between your thumb and index finger about the width of your hand from the top of the page (see fig. 3.1). When your partner drops the paper, catch it before it slips through the thumb and finger. There is no numerical score in this activity: It's pass or fail. Do not move hand lower to catch paper.

5. **On your mark** (speed)
   Time children in a 40-yard sprint. Use two cones to mark the distance.

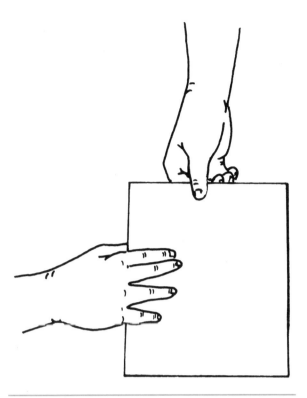

Fig. 3.1. *Gravity grab*

6. **Off the wall** (coordination)
   Standing four feet from a wall, throw underhand and catch a tennis ball against the wall alternating hands. Students crouch, lean forward slightly, and use an underhand catch. The score is number of catches in 30 seconds.

Discuss how these skill-fitness components are necessary for success in sports. Use the following descriptions to discuss components.

Cool-Down: 5 Minutes

Select stretching and cool-down activities.

Skill-Fitness Descriptions

Arrange students in partners to discuss and list sports or activities in which each of the following skills are important. Share with the whole class and list on chart paper.

Balance—maintaining body control while stationary or moving, for example, ice skating or tumbling

Power—moving a weight or the body as quickly as possible, for example, throwing a discus or weight lifting

Agility—changing direction of the body quickly and smoothly, for example, snow skiing or a running back in football

Reaction time—the time between hearing a sound and moving the body, for example, sprint start in running or swimming

Speed—moving the entire body as rapidly as possible over a short distance, for example, 100-yard sprint

Coordination—the ability to use the body to catch, kick, or hit a ball, for example, playing basketball and soccer

Teaching Tips

Let the students have one practice attempt at each activity.

Ask students to develop a poem using the following as an example:

Line 1—One word that names exercise or activity.

Line 2—Two words that tell how the first word looks or moves.

Line 3—Three words that tell about the first word.

Line 4—Two words that tell something special about the first word.

Line 5—One word same as line one.

Example

1 word—push-ups
2 words—building strength
3 words—straining vertical motion
2 words—makes muscles
1 words—push-ups

Handout 3.1   Skill Fitness Score Sheet

Name_____

Date_____

Directions: Complete your score for each test item.

Component	Activity	Score
1. Balance	Stork stand	_____ Seconds
2. Power	Blast off	_____ Inches
3. Agility	Chair slalom	_____ Seconds
4. Reaction time	Gravity grab	Pass/Fail
5. Speed	On your mark	_____ Seconds
6. Coordination	Off the wall	_____ Number

WEEK 3

Lesson 12

Health Fitness

Goals

- To understand the components of health-related fitness
- To measure health-related fitness of each student

Key Concepts

Cardiovascular endurance, low-back and thigh flexibility, muscular endurance, and body composition are components of health-related fitness. An acceptable level of health-related fitness helps to prevent disease and other ailments later in life.

Cardiovascular endurance—ability to exercise the body continuously over long periods. Refers to fitness of the heart, lungs, and blood vessels.

Flexibility—range of motion of a joint and muscle groups around the joint, for example, reaching down to touch the toes stretches the back and the back of the leg muscles.

Muscular endurance—ability to use muscles many times without becoming tired, for example, stomach muscles during sit-ups.

Body composition (body fatness)—body composition refers to the amount of muscle, bone, and fat in the body. Too much body fat (over 30 percent) causes a health risk. Fat develops in the body when a person takes in more calories than they are using in daily activities. Food contains calories, and energy from calories is essential for life. For every extra pound of fat a person carries, the heart must pump blood through an extra mile of blood vessels.

Materials

1. Stopwatch
2. Sit-and-reach box or yardstick (or measuring tape), masking tape
3. Mats
4. Handout 3.2 Health Fitness Score Sheet

Brainstorm ideas with your class about the benefits of being physically fit.

- Feel good (not tired all the time)
- Be strong (able to do physical work)
- Enjoy recreational activities (bicycling, swimming, sports, skiing)
- Stay healthy (reduce risk of health problems related to lack of exercise)
- Sleep better
- Live longer
- Increased energy for learning

Warm-Up: 5 Minutes

Select stretching and warm-up activities.

Activity: Health Fitness

The lesson consists of four fitness tests. Students record their scores on handout 3.2.

1. **Mile or half-mile run** (cardiovascular endurance)
   Based on the time and facilities available, select either a half-mile or a mile timed run. A mile is preferable because children will exercise for a longer time, thus making it more of an endurance activity. However, this may take an extra lesson.
2. **Sit and reach** (flexibility)
   Use a sit-and-reach box (see fig. 3.2), yardstick, or measuring tape. If using a yardstick or measuring tape, put a piece of masking tape on the floor. Sit perpendicular to it with your legs extended, knees straight, heels five to seven inches apart and just touching the inside edge of the tape. Place a yardstick or measuring tape between your legs, with the 15-inch mark on the inside edge of the tape. A partner holds your knees straight. Place hands one on top of the other with all fingers matching. Reach forward with both hands as far as possible and touch the stick. Record the score to the nearest half inch. The score is the best of three trials.
3. **Sit-ups** (muscular endurance)
   Student lies on back with knees flexed and feet flat on the floor. Heels are between 12 and 18 inches from the buttocks. The arms are crossed on the chest with the hands on opposite shoulders. A partner holds the feet

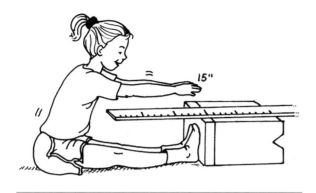

Fig. 3.2. Sit-and-reach box

to keep them in contact with the ground. The student curls to the sitting position. Maintain arm contact with the chest. Keep the chin tucked on the chest. The sit-up is completed when the elbows touch the thighs. The student returns to the down position in which the midback contacts the surface of the mat. The score is the number of completed sit-ups in 60 seconds.

4. **Pinch test** (body composition)
   Children pinch their bodies in three places to feel the amount of fat beneath the skin. The three places are on the back of the upper arm above the elbow, at the hip, and on the front of the thigh. Tell the students to try to determine for themselves whether they have a lot of fat, some fat, or a little fat. This is subjective and does not translate into a score. It does, however, raise awareness levels. You can do an accurate skinfold measurement with calipers.

Cool-Down: 5 Minutes

Select stretching and cool-down activities.

Teaching Tips

Children can work in pairs and take turns testing each other and recording scores. Students will obviously compare scores. There is a need to emphasize that scores are a baseline measure and individual improvement is the goal. Students can be retested periodically throughout the year and you can chart progress.

Handout 3.2   Health Fitness Score Sheet

Name_____

	Run	Sit and reach	Sit-ups

Test 1

Date: _____   _____   _____   _____

Test 2

Date: _____   _____   _____   _____

Test 3

Date: _____   _____   _____   _____

Test 4

Date: _____   _____   _____   _____

WEEK 3

Lesson 13

Skill Stops

Goals

- To reinforce skill-related fitness activities and concepts
- To improve coordination, reaction time, speed, power, agility, and balance skills

Key Concepts

Station activities allow practice of sport skills that help develop skill-related fitness. This organizational approach permits intensive practice on selected sports skills.

Materials

1. Cones
2. Four soccer balls
3. Six basketballs or playground balls
4. One softball
5. One Frisbee
6. Three footballs
7. One volleyball
8. One playground ball

Warm-Up: 5 Minutes

Select stretching and warm-up activities.

Activity: Skill Stops

- Divide class into groups of three or four.
- Organize six stations (from the eight examples) that emphasize sport skills (see fig. 3.3).
- All skill stops contain elements of each skill-related fitness component.
- Allow two or three minutes at each station.

1. **Soccer dribble:** Set up a square 10 × 10 yards with cones.
   As soon as the first player reaches cone three, the next player can go.
2. **Basketball rebound:** Use a hoop and backboard.
   Player 1 dribbles to the free throw line and shoots. Player 2 rebounds the ball and passes it to player 3, who shoots. Player 4 rebounds

the ball and passes it to player 1. Players 1 and 2, and 3 and 4 change roles next time through.
3. **Basketball dribble and shoot:** Use a hoop and backboard.
   Player 1 dribbles in and out of the cones, shoots, retrieves the ball, and goes to the end of the line. When player 1 reaches the last cone the next player can go.
4. **Softball throw and run, catch and run:** Set up a 10 × 10 yard square with cones.
   Player 1 throws the ball to either player 2 or 3 and moves to the vacant corner of the square (use cones). Next player throws to one of the others and moves to vacant cone. Start with a 10 × 10 yard square and increase size according to skill.
5. **Frisbee in the middle:** Set up 12 × 15 yard area with cones.
   Player 1 throws the Frisbee to player 2. Player 3 tries to intercept. Player 1 and 2 can move sideways. Switch positions when the Frisbee is intercepted.
6. **Football zigzag:** Set up a zigzag course with cones.
   Player 1, holding the football, runs in a zigzag pattern in and out of cones. When player 1 reaches the third cone the next player can start. When all three players reach one end they perform the same activity coming back through the cones.
7. **Volleyball passing:** Pass and move in groups of three in a 10-yard space.
   Player 1 volleys or serves the ball to player 3 and follows pass to move behind player 3. Player 3 passes to player 2 and follows pass. Start with throws, then volleyball passing.
8. **Handball rally:** Use a wall and playground ball.
   Players 1, 2, and 3 take turns serving the playground ball against the wall with their hands or fists. Allow any number of bounces.

Cool-Down: 5 Minutes

Select stretching and cool-down activities.

Skill Stops

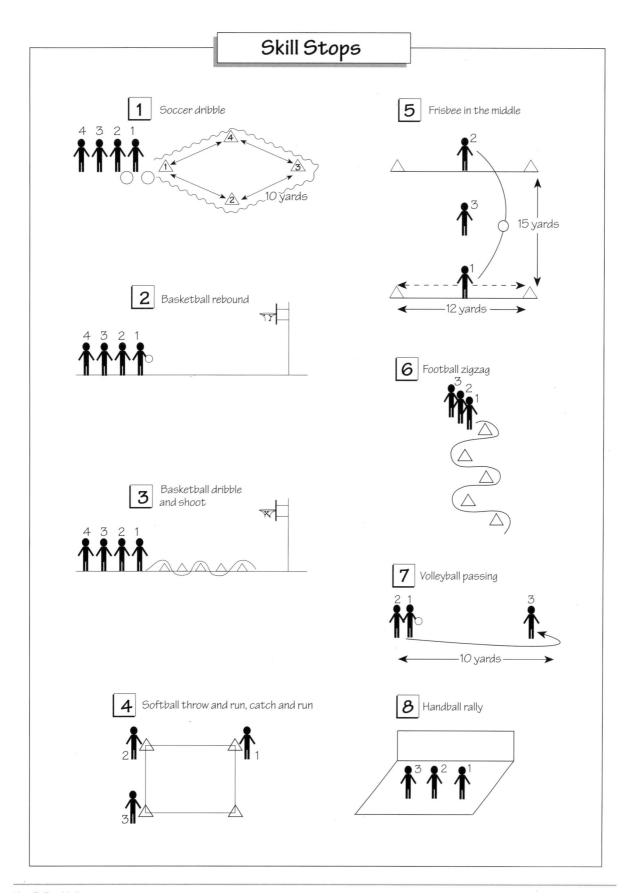

Fig. 3.3. Skill stops

Teaching Tips

At end of the lesson during cool-down, help children identify the skill-related fitness components in each sport activity. All the components are needed to a certain extent, but some will occur in greater amounts. For example, the handball rally primarily requires coordination, but additional components are needed to a lesser extent. It is helpful to have task cards at each station. Reinforce what skill-fitness components you are measuring. You can do this lesson indoors. If so, clearly define each activity area and reduce dimensions if necessary.

WEEK 3

Lesson 14

Fitness Fortune

Goal

- To improve cardiovascular endurance, strength, and flexibility

Key Concepts

Fitness levels improve with regular practice and when students push themselves a little harder each time to improve. A gradual increase in intensity is an essential principle. The "no pain, no gain" adage is often counterproductive because pain can signify injury, which prevents participation in exercise programs.

Materials

1. Thirty-two strips of paper with one activity written on each
2. Jump ropes (eight–10)
3. Mats

Warm-Up: 5 Minutes

Select stretching and warm-up activities.

Activity: Fitness Fortune

- Before class write a variety of endurance activities on individual strips of paper (about 32).

- Fold pieces of paper and place them in center of gym.
- On signal, students pick up one piece of paper, and complete the exercise.
- When finished, students return the folded paper and take another.

Fitness Activities

- Touch every wall in gym without touching a person.
- Jog around gym twice without touching a person.
- Do 30 jumping jacks.
- Do six sit-ups or push-ups in each corner of gym.
- Jump rope 30 times any style.
- Be a judge, walk around gym, and tell three students they are doing a great job.

Use exercises from chapter 13 for other activities.

Cool-Down: 5 Minutes

Select stretching and cool-down activities.

Teaching Tips

Demonstrate and clearly explain each activity. Laminate the strips of paper for future use. Designate areas for each activity. Post signs if necessary.

Lesson 15

Fat Is Where It's At—Not!

Goal

- To introduce the concept that dietary fat and cholesterol may clog blood vessels with fatty deposits

Key Concepts

Foods high in saturated fat and cholesterol may contribute to high blood cholesterol levels, which cause fatty buildup in the arteries called *atherosclerosis*. Narrowed blood vessels force the heart to pump hard, which can lead to heart disease. Cholesterol is not a fat but rather a fat-like material found in the body cells of humans and animals. Animal products contain cholesterol, plant products do not. Not all cholesterol comes from the food we eat. Our liver manufactures cholesterol from saturated fats in our diet and uses it to form cell membranes and hormones. The problem occurs when we consume too much cholesterol and saturated fat in our diet, resulting in a rise of cholesterol levels in the blood. A diet high in saturated fat and cholesterol can lead to a buildup in the blood vessels called *plaque*. Plaque clogs the arteries and prevents the blood from flowing from the heart to the lungs and other tissues. This plaque buildup may begin early in life and continue through adulthood.

Materials

1. Fig. 3.4 Atherosclerosis
2. Handout 3.3 Cholesterol and Saturated Fats in Foods (one per student)
3. About five inches of clear plastic tubing (can be purchased from any hardware, craft, or aquarium store)
4. Two-inch segment of paper towel tubes per group
5. Clay for each group
6. Handout 3.4 Week 3, Family Activity: Home Fitness Stations (one per student)

Activity: Fat Is Where It's At—Not!

- Before class, place a small amount of colored clay inside the clear plastic tubing to simulate plaque.
- Using fig. 3.4, describe what is meant by plaque and what substances are found in the plaque (cholesterol and saturated fat). When a blood clot is lodged in a clogged artery, the flow of blood is halted, resulting in a heart attack. Ask the students what foods they think contain these two substances (cholesterol and saturated fats), and write them on the board (see handout 3.3).
- Provide each student with handout 3.3 and show the class which foods are high in these fatty substances if they are unsure.
- Pass out the segments of paper towel tubing and clay to each student.
- Have students mold plaque in the tube. Instruct certain groups to simulate the different stages of atherosclerosis, from slight to complete blockage.
- Discuss their completed arteries.

Teaching Tips

Instead of colored clay, you could use jello to simulate plaque in the plastic tubing.

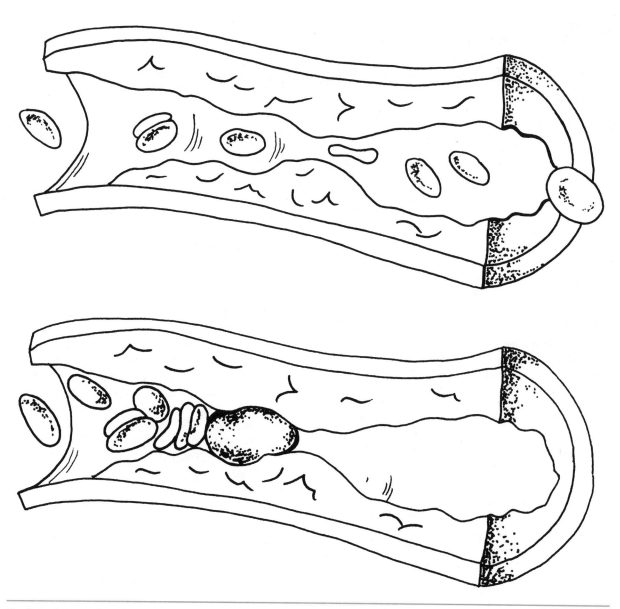

Fig. 3.4. Atherosclerosis

Handout 3.3   Cholesterol and Saturated Fats in Foods

Cholesterol foods

Beef
Cream cheese
Chicken
Cheddar cheese
Fish
Egg yolk
Pork
Butter
Shrimp
Lard

Saturated fats

Butter
Stick margarine
Meats and poultry
Cocoa butter
Sandwich meats
Coconut oil
Whole milk products
Palm oil
Ice cream
Lard or shortening
Egg yolks

Handout 3.4   Week 3, Family Activity: Home Fitness Stations

Select five exercises to use in a family fitness station course at home. Choose exercises ranging from easy to difficult, but select exercises that family members can successfully complete. Use this station sheet and diagram the sequence of the exercises. Set up the five stations in the house or yard. The objective is to complete three circuits of each station. Select the number of repetitions at each station. Start with a low number (two-four) of repetitions at each station.

1. Names of family members

_____

_____

2. Describe exercises

    Exercise 1 _____

    Exercise 2 _____

    Exercise 3 _____

    Exercise 4 _____

    Exercise 5 _____

3. Diagram sequence of exercises.

4. Record the dates and repetitions for each family member for one week.

5. Ask family members to write a short comment about this activity. Family members can comment on enjoyment level, exertion level, if they would continue to do it regularly.

Time: 45 minutes

Please return by _____.

CHAPTER 4

Week 4: Risk Factors

The lessons introduce the concept of inheriting specific biological traits and lifestyles that contribute to cardiovascular disease. The nutrition information explains the Food Pyramid and relates it to daily food choices.

WEEK 4

Lesson 16

What Are Risk Factors?

Goals

- To introduce the concept of risk factors for heart disease
- To help students understand that some risk factors can be controlled and some cannot

Key Concepts

Risk factors are circumstances or lifestyle habits that increase the risk of acquiring heart disease. This lesson points out that lifestyles have changed and some of those changes put us at risk for heart disease.

Materials

Handout 4.1 Risk Factor Checklist

Activity: What Are Risk Factors?

Discuss differences between life in earlier times (1800s) and life now. Talk about how life has changed in terms of daily living and discuss how some of the outcomes are decreased physical activity and changes in diet. Develop a list with two columns that shows how things have changed.

Life long ago

Physical chores (cutting wood, growing food)

Walk to school

Little transportation

No electric appliances

Hand tools (often bones from animals)

Life now

Fewer physical chores (going to the store to buy food)

Ride bus to school

Extensive transportation

Gas and electric-powered machines do most of the work

Use the following questions to help children brainstorm their lists:

- How do families obtain food, prepare, and save it?
- How do they find shelter and obtain clothing?
- Where do they get water for washing and drinking?
- How do they get from place to place?
- Did people living in the 1800s exercise more or less than people today? Why?
- What inventions have led to a society in which people exercise less?
- What can people do today to ensure getting adequate exercise?

Point out that improvements in health care such as vaccinations have enabled people to live longer. The danger now is not from infectious diseases, but from our own lifestyle. Present the following as risk factors for heart disease: inactivity, obesity, high blood pressure, smoking, stress and tension, cholesterol and fatty foods, heredity, gender, age.

Use the Risk Factor Checklist in handout 4.1 to help children examine the risks that they can control and those that they cannot control.

Explanation of risk factors

Age—age is a risk factor for heart disease because other factors, such as a poor diet, lack of exercise, and obesity, are more likely to exist in older persons.

Inactivity—children and adults need to participate in activities that are vigorous enough to improve cardiovascular endurance. Lack of exercise and sitting in front of television leads to an inactive lifestyle. Inactivity may lead to increased weight as well as poor physical fitness.

Obesity—children and adults with high amounts of body fat are at a greater risk for heart disease. The heart has to work hard to pump blood through a body with many fat cells. Children who carry extra weight do not feel comfortable or confident in physical activities and are often easily fatigued.

High blood pressure—there are some 60,000 miles of blood vessels running through the body. As the heart forces the blood through these vessels, the blood is under pressure. Blood pressure is a measure of force exerted against the walls of the blood vessels. Blood pressure is measured in millimeters of mercury and expressed in two numbers. Normal blood pressure is 120/80 or below: The higher number reflects the pressure exerted during the forceful contraction of the heart and the lower number during the heart's relaxation phase. The American Heart Association considers all blood pressures over 140/90 as high. This level of pressure damages the blood vessels.

Smoking—cigarettes contain nicotine that damages the insides of the blood vessels and increases blood pressure. Smoking cigarettes has been strongly linked to lung cancer. It also causes shortness of breath and fatigue.

Stress and tension—fear, anxiety, frustration, fatigue, and hostility increase heart rate and blood pressure. In turn, the heart and blood vessels are adversely affected by the chemicals and hormones the body produces under stress.

Cholesterol and fatty foods—everyone needs to have some cholesterol. In fact our bodies depend on it to form cells and hormones. But, when we eat too many foods rich in cholesterol and fats, cholesterol builds up in our blood stream. It can form a thick, hard coating on the inner walls of blood vessels, reducing blood flow to the heart and brain and increasing the risk of heart attack.

Gender—men are much more likely to develop cardiovascular disease than women.

Heredity—children inherit characteristics from their parents. If parents have heart disease, there is a chance heart disease will be passed on to their children.

Teaching Tips

Children may want to interview their grandparents to gain a better perspective on how life has changed during this century.

Handout 4.1.   Risk Factor Checklist

Name_____

	Cannot control	Can control	How?
Age	_____	_____	_____
Inactivity	_____	_____	_____
Obesity	_____	_____	_____
High blood pressure	_____	_____	_____
Smoking	_____	_____	_____
Stress and tension	_____	_____	_____
Cholesterol and fatty foods	_____	_____	_____
Gender	_____	_____	_____
Heredity	_____	_____	_____

Write a paragraph outlining your strengths and weaknesses in relation to the risk factors. Describe any proposed lifestyle changes.

WEEK 4

Lesson 17

9-1-1 Tag Game

Goals

- To recognize heart attack symptoms and know what to do in an emergency
- To know proper procedures to take in an emergency
- To improve cardiovascular endurance

Key Concepts

Adults with heart disease may be unaware of their likelihood of a heart attack. Due to disease, the heart may be unable to function and a heart attack may occur.

Heart attack symptoms include uncomfortable pressure or pain in the center of the chest lasting more than few minutes; pain spreading to the shoulders, neck, or arms; and chest discomfort with lightheadedness, fainting, sweating, nausea, or shortness of breath.

Materials

1. Two or three Nerf balls
2. Six to eight cones

Warm-Up: 5 Minutes

Select stretching and warm-up activities.

Activity: 9-1-1 Tag Game

- Explain the procedures to call 911 (only in an emergency): State address, describe situation, stay on line, follow directions from 911 operator.

- Mark out a playing area the size of a basketball court with cones.
- Before beginning the activity, briefly present heart attack symptoms and procedure for calling 911.
- Select two or three taggers, who try to touch students with Nerf balls between the shoulder and waist.
- When a player is tagged for the first time, he or she continues to play holding their left arm above the elbow with right hand.
- When tagged a second time, players grasp their chest with both hands.
- When a player is tagged a third time, players freeze, grab throat, and shout "911!"
- They are freed by completing 10 jumping jacks with a player who has not been tagged.

Cool-Down: 5 Minutes

Select stretching and cool-down activities.

Teaching Tips

Change exercise for players who have "heart attacks." Reinforce the concept that exercise helps make a healthy and strong heart. Change taggers every two minutes. Specific medications given immediately after a heart attack can help to dissolve blood clots in arteries and restore blood flow. For a variation, two students could act as blood clot dissolving medications, Streptokinase or TPA, and rescue players having a heart attack. Rescuers and heart attack victims complete 10 repetitions of an exercise together.

Lesson 18

Risky Business

Goal

- To distinguish risk factors that can be controlled from those that can't be controlled

Key Concepts

Risk factors are divided into two categories—those you can control (inactivity, cholesterol, fatty foods, smoking, stress) and those you can't control (age, gender, heredity). Emphasize education programs about developing a lifestyle that promotes physical activity and a heart-healthy diet.

Materials

Three sets of cards with risk factors and exercises

Warm-Up: 5 Minutes

Select stretching and warm-up activities.

Activity: Risky Business

- Divide class into groups of three. Spread each group out in a circle within the playing area.
- The teacher has a group of cards with the name of a risk factor and an exercise routine.
- One student from each group runs to get a card from the teacher and returns to the group.

- The group completes the exercise routine and determines whether or not the risk factor is controllable. If it is controllable, they keep the card and another group member runs to pick up a new card. This continues until each group receives all of the controllable risk factor cards.
- If a group receives a card they think is a noncontrollable risk factor, all group members complete the exercise, jog the outside of the gym or playground, returning to their original place, and return the card to the teacher.
- The objective is to gain all the controllable risk factor cards. When a group collects all these cards, they stand one behind the other in a straight line with their hands in the air.

Cool-Down: 5 Minutes

Select stretching and cool-down activities.

Teaching Tips

Use the exercises in chapter 13 to write out exercises and name of risk factors on cards and laminate. Specify the number of repetitions for each exercise. Make three sets of cards. Use familiar exercises, such as mountain climbers, crab kicks, sit-ups, and push-ups. To provide variety, include cards with one or two repetitions and some cards that require many (25–30) repetitions.

Lesson 19

Seven-Five-Three

Goals

- To develop cardiovascular and muscular endurance
- To find a winning formula for Seven-Five-Three mathematical challenge

Key Concepts

Seven-Five-Three is a mathematical puzzle with rows of seven, five, and three sticks. Students are challenged to play with a partner and solve the puzzle.

Materials

Fifteen Popsicle sticks or cards for each pair with names of exercises written on sticks or cards. (For a class of 30 students, 225 sticks are required.)

Warm-Up: 5 Minutes

Select stretching and warm-up activities.

Activity: Seven-Five-Three

- To play the game of Seven-Five-Three, use three rows of Popsicle sticks or cards (see fig. 4.1), with the printed side face down.
- Students take turns picking up the sticks.
- You can only pick up one or two Popsicle sticks. However many you chose, they must all be from the same row.
- The student picking up the stick(s) performs the exercise written on them.
- The other student runs to touch each wall of the gym or around designated cones while the partner performs the exercise.
- The winner is the student who forces his or her partner to pick up the last stick from the remaining pile.

Cool-Down: 5 Minutes

Select stretching and cool-down activities.

Teaching Tips

Students in pairs make sticks in class and band sets together. Write the names of exercises on each Popsicle stick. Use exercises from chapter 13. Tell students to touch walls with their hands and to slow down before touching the wall. Establish guidelines to avoid collision.

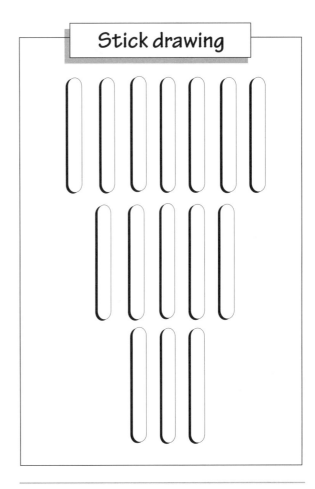

Fig. 4.1. *Seven-five-three*

Lesson 20

The Final Four Plus Two

Goals

- To introduce the Food Pyramid
- To emphasize the importance of a balanced diet

Key Concepts

In 1956, the basic four food groups were devised to promote the health of all Americans. The problem with the groupings is that it appears to place greater emphasis on animal products higher in fat (i.e., meat and dairy) than those food groups high in carbohydrates and low in fat (grains, vegetables, and fruits). The Food Pyramid was therefore designed by the USDA as a daily guide to emphasize a high carbohydrate, low-fat approach to eating. The new pyramid retains the four food groups but emphasizes the importance of grains, fruits, and vegetables, which don't contain fat and cholesterol.

To be fit requires eating a balanced diet of carbohydrates, protein, fat, vitamins, minerals, and water. Most foods contain various combinations of these nutrients. The Food Pyramid helps guide you in the kinds and amounts of foods to eat every day. There are six blocks in the pyramid.

   a. Bread, cereal, rice, and pasta—6 to 11 servings; 1 serving is equal to 1 slice of bread or 1/2 cup of cereal, rice, or pasta.

   b. Vegetables—3 to 5 servings each day; 1 serving equals 1/2 cup.

   c. Fruit—2 to 4 servings each day; 1 serving equals a small orange, 1/2 banana, or 1/2 cup chopped fruit.

   d. Milk, yogurt, and cheese (milk group)—2 or 3 servings per day; 1 serving equals 1 cup or 8 ounces of milk or yogurt or 1 ounce of cheese.

   e. Meat, poultry, fish, dry beans, eggs, and nuts—2 or 3 servings per day; 1 serving equals 1 ounce of meat, 1/3 cup of beans, 1 egg, or 2 tablespoons of nuts.

   f. Fats, oils, and sweets are the smallest block—0 or 1 serving (sparingly) or once in a while; a serving equals 1 teaspoon of margarine or 1 teaspoon of sugar.

Materials

1. Fig. 4.2, basic four food group plan (one per student)
2. Fig. 4.3, food pyramid (one per student)
3. A set of building blocks, figs. 4.4 (one copy per group), 4.5 (2 copies per group), 4.6 (three copies per group). Copy each building block and enlarge on the copier as needed.
4. Scissors and glue per group.
5. Handout 4.2 Week 4, Family Activity: Media Watch (one per student)

Activity: The Final Four Plus Two

- Brainstorm with the students.
  a. What do you know about the basic four food groups? The Food Pyramid?
  b. What do you need to know?
  c. How do we find out?
- Using the answers to these questions, review the information about basic four food groups and introduce the Food Pyramid.
- Hand out the building block templates. Before cutting them out, ask the students to
  a. write the name of the food group on each block (according to the size of the blocks), and
  b. list the types of foods in each group.
- Cut out and construct pyramid.
- After the pyramid has been built, ask, "What would happen if you removed the dairy group?" (The pyramid would fall apart.) "Which building block could you remove without destroying the pyramid?" (the fats, oils, and sweets group)
- Conclude the lesson by brainstorming, "What did you learn?" with the students.

Teaching Tips

Templates should be copied onto heavier paper, preferably different colors. You could read *Cloudy With a Chance of Meatballs* by Judi Berrett as an introduction to this lesson. Give each group a Ziploc bag to store their pyramids for later use. You can provide additional templates to each student for homework. Ask the students to begin collecting empty food packages, labels, photographs, signs, and slogans that convey healthy eating habits and bring them to class for future lessons. Begin collecting reference materials that list the nutritional content of various fast food for use in lesson 30.

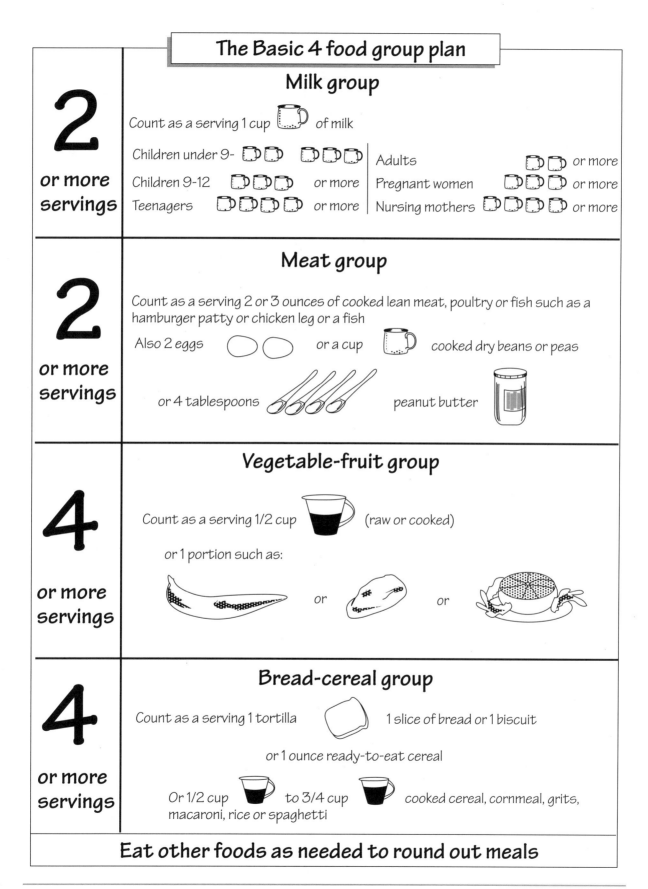

The Basic 4 food group plan

Milk group

2 or more servings

Count as a serving 1 cup of milk

Children under 9-	Adults — or more
Children 9-12 — or more	Pregnant women — or more
Teenagers — or more	Nursing mothers — or more

Meat group

2 or more servings

Count as a serving 2 or 3 ounces of cooked lean meat, poultry or fish such as a hamburger patty or chicken leg or a fish

Also 2 eggs   or a cup   cooked dry beans or peas

or 4 tablespoons   peanut butter

Vegetable-fruit group

4 or more servings

Count as a serving 1/2 cup   (raw or cooked)

or 1 portion such as:

Bread-cereal group

4 or more servings

Count as a serving 1 tortilla   1 slice of bread or 1 biscuit

or 1 ounce ready-to-eat cereal

Or 1/2 cup   to 3/4 cup   cooked cereal, cornmeal, grits, macaroni, rice or spaghetti

Eat other foods as needed to round out meals

Fig. 4.2. Basic four food group plan

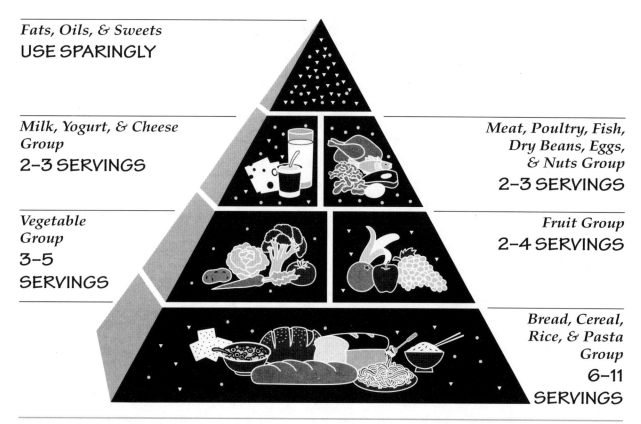

Fats, Oils, & Sweets
USE SPARINGLY

Milk, Yogurt, & Cheese Group
2–3 SERVINGS

Meat, Poultry, Fish, Dry Beans, Eggs, & Nuts Group
2–3 SERVINGS

Vegetable Group
3–5 SERVINGS

Fruit Group
2–4 SERVINGS

Bread, Cereal, Rice, & Pasta Group
6–11 SERVINGS

Fig. 4.3. Food pyramid

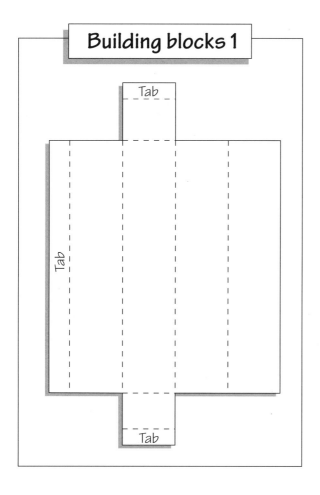

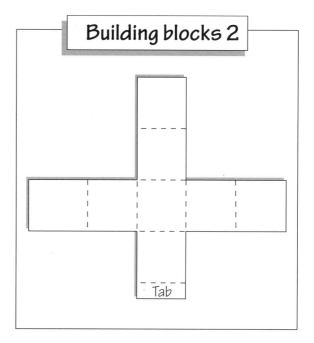

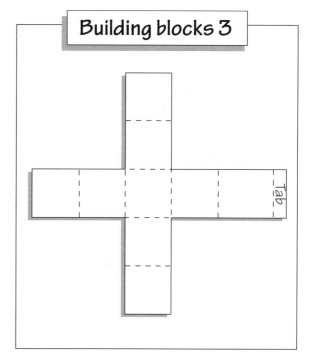

Fig. 4.4–4.6. Building blocks

Handout 4.2   Week 4, Family Activity: Media Watch

Watch television with your family members on Saturday morning, paying special attention to commercials. Have a family discussion and complete the following questions.

1. What kinds of food products were advertised?

2. What was your favorite food advertisement?

   Why?

3. Why does the commercial say you should buy the product? (e.g., it is fortified, will make you grow big and strong)

4. Is the product supported by a favorite personality (movie star, sports figure, cartoon character)?

   Who?

5. Do you think the food product is good for you?

6. Does the advertisement make you want to buy the product?

7. Would you buy a product because you liked the commercial?

   Why or why not?

Time: 30 minutes

Please return by _____.

Week 5: Aerobic Fitness

The lessons introduce taking pulse rates and the activity segments provide opportunities to develop this skill. Students learn about serving sizes and how to measure quantities of food.

WEEK 5

Lesson 21

The Beat Goes On

Goals

- To find and record a pulse rate
- To compare resting, peak, and cool-down pulse rates

Key Concepts

Students learn how physical exercise affects the cardiovascular system. The pulse rate is the best indicator of physical exertion levels and is relatively easy to monitor. The pulse rate reflects how hard the heart is working. Resting pulse rates are lower in persons with high levels of physical fitness.

Materials

1. Handout 5.1 The Beat Goes On (one per student)
2. Handout 5.2 Week 5, Family Activity: The Beat Goes Home (one per student)

Activity: The Beat Goes On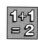

- The pulse rate is the number of times the heart pumps each minute. This rate changes with your activity level. When you're calm and relaxed, your pulse is called "resting" and is slower. When you are active, scared, or excited it is at a "peak" and the heart pumps faster increasing the pulse rate.
- When you were born, your pulse was about 130 to 140 beats per minute. As you grew, your pulse rate slowed gradually to 80 to 90 beats per minute in childhood. It is even slower for an adult, 70 to 80 beats per minute. Boys often have a lower pulse rate because a boy's heart is slightly larger than a girl's heart.
- Hard exercise causes your pulse rate to increase rapidly. Most of the increase occurs in the first two minutes. After that, it increases gradually and levels off. When the exercise stops, your pulse rate may take two to five minutes to return to normal.

First Activity

Finding your pulse rate (Provide Handout 5.1 The Beat Goes On.)

- Place your index and middle fingers on your neck (carotid artery) or wrist in line with the thumb (radial artery). Don't use your thumb for taking the pulse rate because the pulse in your thumb may interfere with your count (see fig. 5.1).
- Hold your fingers in place until you feel the steady beat of your pulse.
- Count the beats for six seconds. Multiply this count by 10 to find the number of beats per minute. Record number under "resting rate." As a backup, count for a minute and compare to the six-second count method.
- Repeat the previous step at least three times. Be available to help students find their pulse rate.

Second Activity

- Bring students outdoors or to gymnasium for five minutes of exercise or jogging to increase pulse rate. Remember to conduct a warm-up routine.
- Immediately afterward, have students find and count their pulse for six seconds. Multiply by 10 to determine beats per minute—record peak rate.
- After walking for one minute, find and record the cool-down pulse rate, reinforcing

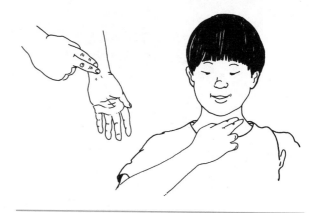

Fig. 5.1. Taking a pulse

the concept of cool-down, meaning the rate at which their exertion level has cooled or slowed following exercise.

- Return to the classroom, record the peak and cool-down pulse rates.
- Encourage students to practice finding their pulse rate at home during all types of activities, including when they are resting or watching TV. Have the students complete the remainder of the chart as homework and return it to school.
- Each student can graph their individual pulse rate profile.
- This lesson reprinted with permission from the July/August issue of *Learning91,* copyright © 1991, Springhouse Corporation, 1111 Bethlehem Pike, Springhouse, PA 19477. All rights reserved.

Teaching Tips

For extra math practice ask students to complete the following. If your heart beats once per second, how many times does it beat in a minute, hour, day, week, month, year, decade? Have each student take their pulse rate. Using the scores of each class member, introduce frequencies. Students can bar or line graph the results. Discuss how individual heart rates vary between students and that exercise can help lower heart rates.

Handout 5.1   The Beat Goes On (Finding Your Pulse Rate)

1. Place index and middle fingers on your wrist (radial) or neck (carotid). Don't use your thumb because the pulse in your thumb may interfere with your count.

2. Hold your fingers in place until you feel the steady beat of your pulse.

3. Count the beats for six seconds. Multiply this count by 10 to find the number of beats per minute.

   6 seconds × 10 = 60 seconds or 1 minute

4. My resting pulse is _____.

Heart chart

	Date	Activity	Pulse	Classification
1.	_____	jogging in place	_____	P
2.	_____	walking	_____	C
3.	_____	_____	_____	_____
4.	_____	_____	_____	_____
5.	_____	_____	_____	_____
6.	_____	_____	_____	_____

Classification key

R = Resting
W = Warm-up
P = Peak
C = Cool-down

Handout 5.2   Week 5, Family Activity: The Beat Goes Home

This activity teaches a family member how to take a pulse rate. The family member can take his or her pulse rate while resting or sitting down. Then the family member can retake his or her pulse rate during light activity, such as walking. Record the pulse rates of the family member during different activities.

Family member_____

Resting pulse rate_____

Activity	Pulse rate
1. _____	_____
2. _____	_____
3. _____	_____
4. _____	_____
5. _____	_____
6. _____	_____
7. _____	_____
8. _____	_____

Time: 40 to 60 minutes.

Please return by _____.

WEEK 5

Lesson 22

Target Practice

Goals

- To identify a target rate for each student
- To learn to increase an activity level to reach target heart rate

Key Concepts

A target heart rate represents enough effort to improve the function of the cardiovascular system. Exercising for 15 to 20 minutes at the target heart rate increases the efficiency of the heart muscle and improves the vitality of the cardiovascular system.

Materials

Five cones

Warm-Up: 5 Minutes

Select stretching and warm-up activities.

Activity: Target Practice

To maintain cardiovascular fitness, keep the heart rate in the target zone. The chart below shows when the heart rate is in the target zone for children.

If your resting heart rate is	Target heart rate is
< 60	150
60–64	151
65–69	153
70–74	155
75–79	157
80–84	159
85–89	161
90>	163

Use the following workout activities to help your children monitor their heart rate. Before starting the activity have the children take a resting pulse (see lesson 21).

Activity 1: Run around the leader

- Divide class into groups of three to five students.
- Instruct teams to follow their leader in a slow jog wherever the leader goes (leaders should not run in circles).
- At a whistle signal, the last student in formation sprints around other students until he or she is the new leader. Students must stay in formation, which requires pacing, until each student has sprinted around the leader, at which time the team slowly jogs in place.

Activity 2: Run around the answer

- Students form an inner and outer circle, standing side by side.
- On signal, pairs jog in place, pacing to stay together.
- They exchange answers to a designated question before a signal, at which time the inner partners jog a circuit and stop at the next person forward.
- Questions should relate to content previously taught, for example, what is the name of the blood vessel in the neck used for taking the pulse rate?

Activity 3: Zigzag jog

- Set up cones as shown in fig. 5.2.
- Partner 1 starts at cone A, partner 2 starts at cone D.
- Partners 1 and 2 run to cone B, do a hand slap (high five), then partner 1 runs around cones D and C and back to B.
- Partner 2 runs around cone A and E and back to B for another hand slap.
- From there, partner 1 runs around cone E and ends at cone A.
- Partner 2 runs around cone C and ends at D.
- Once students become familiar with the course, introduce balls they can pass off to one another.
- Encourage a slow to moderate jog, so students don't overtake each other.

Cool-Down: 5 Minutes

Select stretching and cool-down activities.

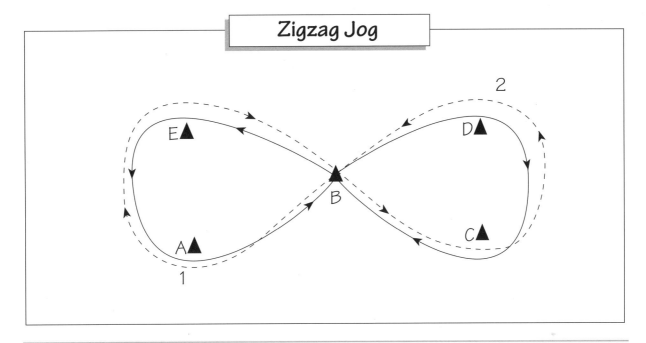

Zigzag Jog

Fig. 5.2. Zigzag jog

Teaching Tips

Children can periodically take their pulse rate. Establish a target heart rate for each student using the table. Students take their resting pulse and identify a target rate. Use the PE scale (from lesson 8) to help students associate their pulse rates with the PE scale. An alternative method (used by adults) of establishing a target heart rate is to subtract their age from 220. Sixty percent of that number is the bottom range of the target rate. Generally, a target pulse rate is 60 to 75 percent of 220 minus age. The following is an example for a 12-year-old child.

220 – 12 = 208
60% of 208 = 125
75% of 208 = 156

The target heart rate for a 12-year-old is 125 (60%) to 156 (75%). The disadvantage of using this method is that it doesn't take resting heart rate into account. Before class students can generate questions for Run Around the Answer.

WEEK 5

Lesson 23
Still Walkin'

Goals

- To introduce a walking workout schedule to children
- To establish a five-week walking program for children and their friends and families

Key Concepts

Walking has considerable lifetime value and is therefore worth introducing to children and their families. Walking is an easy-to-organize activity for children that they can complete with family members.

Materials

1. Popsicle sticks or chips
2. Handout 5.3 Walking Is Super Healthy (WISH) (one per student)

Warm-Up: 5 Minutes

Select stretching and warm-up activities.

Activity: Still Walkin'

- Map out a mile for a class walk. You can use a track or a specific walking course in your school. Students can participate in calculating a mile course.
- The objective for this class lesson is for everyone to walk one mile. If you use a track, use Popsicle sticks or chips to help students keep track of their laps. Clearly explain that this activity is a walk, not a run. Tell the class that in another lesson you will ask them to run. Invite parents to walk with you.
- Use the class walk to establish a five-week walking program for your class.
- Students can form small groups in class. Each group decides on a place in the United States they would like to visit. Use an atlas to find out how far away that destination is.
- Divide the number of miles to the imaginary destination by 15 to determine how many miles each one-mile walk session represents.

For example, a person living in San Francisco that decided to take an imaginary trip to New York would divide the 2,500-mile distance by 15 and discover that each of their workouts represented 167 miles.

- Use the Walking Is Super Healthy chart (handout 5.3) to complete the program.

Cool-Down: 5 Minutes

Select stretching and cool-down activities. Introduce and explain handout 5.3 Walking Is Super Healthy.

Teaching Tips

Students can complete their walking activities at school during recess, breaks, and lunch hour. Ask your students to share their pretend destinations and why these places had special appeal. Then turn your walkers into researchers by having them read about their destinations and report on tourist attractions and other points of interest. Encourage them to provide additional information about some of the locations they could visit en route to their pretend destinations. Parent and school permission is needed for any course off the school grounds.

This lesson reprinted with permission from the July/August issue of *Learning91*, copyright © 1991, Springhouse Corporation, 1111 Bethlehem Pike, Springhouse, PA 19477. All rights reserved.

Handout 5.3   Walking Is Super Healthy (WISH)

Name_____

Destination_____

Miles to Destination_____

"Imaginary Journey Miles" per workout_____

Week	Walk 1	Walk 2	Walk 3	Weekly total
1	_____	_____	_____	_____
2	_____	_____	_____	_____
3	_____	_____	_____	_____
4	_____	_____	_____	_____
5	_____	_____	_____	_____

Decide on a place your group would like to visit: Use an atlas to find out how far away that destination is. Then divide the number of miles to the imaginary destination by 15 to determine how many miles each of your one-mile walks represents. For example, a person living in San Francisco that decided to take an imaginary trip to New York city would divide the 2,500-mile distance by 15 and discover that each of their workouts represented 167 miles.

Lesson 24

Aerobic Relays and Partner Run

Goals

- To improve cardiovascular endurance
- To perform a variety of locomotion skills

Key Concepts

In a traditional physical education class much time is spent standing around in lines or waiting for a turn. Large numbers in a relay team can reduce time spent in activity. Therefore, make teams as small as possible. Relays are most active with teams of two or three players. Small teams also increase contact time with equipment.

Materials

1. Cones
2. Balls (one per group of three)

Warm-Up: 5 Minutes

Select stretching and warm-up activities.

Activity 1: Aerobic Relays

- Divide class into groups of three.
- Use cones for guide points and a high-five slap for exchanging runners.
- Teams follow specific ending procedures, such as sitting or standing in a straight line with arms above head.
- Assign a student judge for each relay.
- Select relay tasks from the following examples.

1. Run to cone and skip back.
2. Gallop to cone and run back.
3. Grapevine shuffle (side stepping, alternating lead foot forward and backward) to cone and run back.
4. Walk backward to cone and jump (two feet) back.
5. Dribble ball to cone and back.

Activity 2: Partner Run

Students pair up with a running partner of similar ability. Set up a course for running depending on your facilities. Explain that this is the first of four sessions. They will start by running together continuously for a three-minute period. Time interval increases by one minute each session. Partner run sessions are included in lessons 27, 28, and 29.

Cool-Down: 5 Minutes

Select stretching and cool-down activities.

Teaching Tips

Emphasize skill and active performance. Give encouragement and praise for following directions. Because being a judge is a prestigious position, rotate judges and relay members each round. Judges assist you to determine relay performance.

Lesson 25

How Do You Measure Up?

Goal

- To identify serving or portion sizes for different foods

Key Concepts

The Food Pyramid is based on serving sizes that provide enough nutrients and calories. Each food group has an amount per serving based on weight or volume. Knowing the amount of each food that represents one serving is an important tool for a healthy lifestyle. The food groups described in the Food Pyramid have serving sizes based on volume or weight.

1. Bread, cereal, rice, pasta group—1 ounce of cold cereal, 1/2 to 3/4 cup cooked cereal, 1/2 cup pasta or rice, or 1 slice of bread equals 1 serving.
2. Vegetable group—1/2 cup cooked vegetables or 1 cup lettuce equals 1 serving.
3. Fruit group—1 small apple or orange, 1/2 cup chopped fruit, 1/2 banana, or 1/2 cup fruit juice equals 1 serving.
4. Dairy group—1 cup of milk, 8 ounces of yogurt, or 1 ounce of cheese equals 1 serving.
5. Meat group—2 or 3 ounces of meat, chicken, or fish, 1-1/2 cups cooked beans, or 1 egg equals 1 serving.
6. Fats, oils, and sugar group—1 teaspoon of margarine, butter, or oil; 1 tablespoon of salad dressing or mayonnaise; or 1 teaspoon of sugar or honey equals 1 serving.

Materials

1. Handout 5.4 How Do You Measure Up? (one per student)
2. Paper bowls, paper plates, and 10-ounce paper cups (one each per group)
3. Six instruction cards, one for each station (laminated)
4. Station setups

Puzzle station—measured foods, one from each food group, labeled A, B, C, D, E, or F. For example, a bowl with three cups of cold cereal, one banana, one egg, one and a half cups of vegetables, one tablespoon margarine, and two cups of milk in a glass. Indicate the amount of each food at the station.

Grains station—an empty box of cereal, a large bowl filled with cereal, a measuring cup, and instruction card.

Vegetable station—two cups of any vegetable in a large bowl (frozen peas or corn work well for this station), a measuring cup, and instruction card.

Fruit station—chopped fruit or canned fruit, drained, in a large bowl (fruit cocktail or chopped fresh fruit), a measuring cup, and instruction card.

Meat station—five or six ounces of lunch meat or salami, a scale that weighs ounces, wax paper, and instruction card.

Milk station—a pitcher of milk, a measuring cup, and instruction card.

Fats, oils, and sugar station—a cube of margarine or butter, measuring spoons, and instruction card.

Activity: How Do You Measure Up?

- Before class, set up the seven stations indicated in the materials section.
- Begin the lesson by reviewing with the students the information learned about The Final Four Plus Two (lesson 20). Do they know what a serving from the dairy group looks like (one cup of fluid milk)?
- Instruct the students to observe the foods at the Puzzle Station. Using handout 5.4, each student should predict and record which of the foods are correct serving sizes and which aren't.
- After predicting, organize students into groups of two or three. Explain the procedures they will follow. Each group will be assigned to a station. After completing the task at the station, each group will move to the next station, until they have completed all activities.
- After all the groups have finished, instruct them to observe the foods at the Puzzle Station again. Do they still agree with their initial predictions? Discuss the results with the class.

Fruit Station

1. Serving sizes of fruit vary. For example, 1/2 banana, 10 grapes, one small apple or orange, or 1/2 cup of chopped fruit equals one serving size.
2. Measure one serving of the fruit at this station into the measuring cup provided.
3. Pour this measured amount onto a paper plate and draw an outline of the portion size. Label "fruit" and indicate the amount.
4. Write down examples of portion sizes for fruit on your handout.
5. Return the fruit to the large bowl at the station and move to the next station.

Dairy Station

1. Milk serving sizes are measured in fluid ounces. One cup or eight fluid ounces of milk or yogurt equals one serving.

2. Measure one serving of milk at this station into the paper cup provided and draw a line around the outside of the cup at the top of the milk line.

3. Write down examples of portion sizes for milk and yogurt on your handout.

4. Pour this amount back into the pitcher and move to the next station.

Meat Station

1. The meat group includes meat, poultry, fish, dried beans, eggs, and nuts. One serving is equal to two or three ounces cooked meat, poultry, or fish; one and a half cups cooked dry beans; four tablespoons peanut butter; two eggs; or one and a half cups of nuts.

2. Measure one serving of meat at this station using the scale provided. Place it on the paper plate and draw a line around the meat. Label and indicate the serving size.

3. Write down examples of portion sizes for this food group on your handout.

4. Replace meat and move to the next station.

Fats, Oils, and Sugar Station

1. One serving of fats, such as margarine or butter, and oils equals one teaspoon. Other fats, such as mayonnaise, are not 100 percent fat and therefore, a serving size equals one tablespoon. Sugar, whether it be white sugar, brown sugar, or honey equals one teaspoon.

2. Measure one serving of margarine at this station and place it on the paper plate. Draw a line on the paper plate around the margarine. Label and indicate the serving size.

3. Write down examples of portion sizes for fats, oils, and sugar on your handout.

4. Replace the margarine and move to the next station.

Grain Station

1. Read the label on the cereal box. What are the two ways in which the serving size is measured?

2. Using the measuring cup, measure out the amount of cereal that equals one serving size.

3. Pour this amount of cereal into the paper bowl provided by your teacher.

4. Mark the level of cereal with a pencil or pen on the inside of the bowl.

5. After you complete the measuring, pour the cereal back into the large bowl at the station.

6. Write on your handout the amount of food that equals a serving size from the following:

   a. bread = one slice
   b. cereal = one ounce
   c. pasta or rice = half cup

7. Move to the next station.

Vegetable Station

1. Usually vegetables are measured using half cup equals one serving. The exception is a vegetable such as lettuce where one cup equals one serving.

2. Measure out one serving of the vegetable using the measuring cup.

3. Pour this measured amount onto a paper plate and draw an outline of the portion size. Label "vegetable" and the amount.

4. Write down examples of portion sizes for vegetables on your handout.

5. Return the vegetable to the large bowl at the station and move to the next station.

Handout 5.4   How Do You Measure Up?

Puzzle Station

	List food	Amount	Prediction (Y/N)	Actual (Y/N)	Difference
A.	_____	_____	___	___	_____
B.	_____	_____	___	___	_____
C.	_____	_____	___	___	_____
D.	_____	_____	___	___	_____
E.	_____	_____	___	___	_____
F.	_____	_____	___	___	_____

List all possible servings.

Station 1

Station 2

Station 3

Station 4

Station 5

Station 6

CHAPTER 6

Week 6: More Aerobic Fitness

The lessons introduce categorization of activities and sports based on criteria for aerobic fitness. Students participate in a developmental approach to running with a gradual increase in the duration of the run.

WEEK 6

Lesson 26

Moving on Air

Goal

• To help children identify physical activities that are aerobic

Key Concepts

Aerobic is a Greek word that means "with air." Aerobic activities are those that require air and through which the heart and lungs become more efficient. Aerobic activities can increase the strength and pumping ability of the heart.

Materials

Handout 6.1 Favorite Physical Activities (one per student)

Activity: Moving on Air

The objective of the lesson is to review different activities and determine which ones are aerobic. Write the name of the following activities on the board in three columns:

A	B	C
Swimming	Baseball	Archery
Bicycling	Football	Golf
Active dancing	Tennis	Driving a car
(folk, aerobic)	Softball	Watching TV
Basketball		

Introduce the following discussion points to illustrate how column A consists of aerobic activities:

1. Exercise and activities that require a great deal of energy and use the large muscles in the body.

2. Exercise and activities that increase your breathing and pulse rate more than others. Review lesson 22 Target Practice.
3. Activities that are continuous rather than stop and start.
4. Exercises and activities that are rhythmic and can be sustained for 20 minutes.
5. Compare column A with activities in columns B and C.

Here is an example to share with your students: Playing a game of baseball would not be 15 to 20 minutes of continuous effort because in baseball a player will run for a few seconds then stop moving. Baseball does use large body muscles, but does not consistently get the pulse rate into the target range. Jogging for 20 minutes requires continuous effort, increases the pulse rate, and uses the leg and arm muscles. Exercise and activities such as jogging for 20 minutes are known as *aerobic*. Use the Favorite Physical Activities sheet (handout 6.1) to help children determine which aerobic activities they enjoy. Tell students to take their pulse rates during certain activities. Teach children to associate higher pulse rates with aerobic activity. Clearly explain that if many of their favorite activities are not aerobic, they should not assign negative feelings. Most physical activities are worthwhile.

Teaching Tips

Use the Greek word "aerobic" to lead into a study of Greece and the importance of physical activity to its culture. Give special emphasis to a study of the Olympics. Ask students to determine which current Olympic events are aerobic.

Handout 6.1   Favorite Physical Activities

Name_____

List your five favorite physical activities.

Activity	C (Continual)	T (Target)	M (Muscles)
1. _____			_____
2. _____			_____
3. _____			_____
4. _____			_____
5. _____			_____

Check the appropriate columns:

C if the activity requires *continual* effort for 15 to 20 minutes,
T if the activity increases your pulse rate into the *target* range for 15 to 20 minutes,
M if the activity uses large body *muscles*, for example, legs and arms.

List the favorite activities that were not aerobic and explain why.

1. _____

2. _____

3. _____

List other activities that are aerobic and explain why.

1. _____

2. _____

3. _____

WEEK 6

Lesson 27

Basketball Jamboree

Goals

- To improve cardiovascular endurance
- To develop cooperation

Key Concepts

Basketball is an example of a lifetime sport, an activity that can be enjoyed throughout one's life. Although many adults may no longer play competitive basketball, many continue to enjoy playing in their driveways, backyards, and parks.

Materials

1. One ball per student
2. Twelve cones

Warm-Up: 5 Minutes

Select stretching and warm-up activities.

Activity: Basketball Jamboree

This lesson is a series of basketball passing and dribbling activities.

Memory pass and run

In a circle of at least five, students begin passing the ball to another student who is not directly next to them. Continue with the same pattern of passing. On command students stop passing and the entire group runs around a cone at least 50 yards away (if outside) designated for that group. Stu-dents return to group and continue the same passing pattern. Add another ball so students are now passing two balls.

Dribble fest

Select four students to act as taggers. The remainder have basketballs and dribble within a defined area (use cones or court lines). Once a dribbler is tagged he or she dribbles around a designated cone outside the playing area and returns to the dribble fest and avoids taggers. Change taggers frequently.

Dribble steal

Students dribble their own balls and try to knock other students' balls away without making any physical contact. Designate two safe zones (basketball keys or use cones). Students can dribble in the safe zones without having their balls knocked away. Students can enter and leave the safe zones as they desire.

Activity: Partner Run

Increase the running interval to four minutes. Refer to lesson 24 for specific instructions.

Cool-Down: 5 Minutes

Select stretching and cool-down activities.

Teaching Tips

Students tag by using two fingers or a foam ball.

Lesson 28

Fitness Challenge I

Goals

- To improve cardiovascular endurance, muscular strength, and endurance
- To set personal goals for each exercise

Key Concepts

Students establish a baseline performance level in specific exercises. Use this to assess improvement in performance. Over time, goal setting provides motivation to improve personal levels of performance. Tracking progress helps keep students motivated and feeling a sense of accomplishment.

Materials

1. Mats
2. Handout 6.2 Fitness Challenge Score Sheet (one per student)

Warm-Up: 5 Minutes

Select stretching and warm-up activities.

Activity: Fitness Challenge I

- Organize students into pairs.
- From the following list of activities establish a challenge program. Ask the students to set their own performance goals. Encourage students to set goals that are reasonable and attainable, yet challenging.
- Encourage students to improve performance, working toward a specific goal.
- Allow one minute for each of the following exercises:
  1. Sit-ups
  2. Side leg raises
  3. Crunches
  4. Line jumps
  5. Mountain climbers
  6. Cross-country skiers

Use the Fitness Challenge Score Sheet (handout 6.2) for students to record the number of repetitions for each exercise. You can add or substitute other exercises for the ones listed.

Activity: Partner Run

Increase the running interval to five minutes. Refer to lesson 24 for specific instructions.

Cool-Down: 5 Minutes

Select stretching and cool-down activities.

Teaching Tips

This is a great time to do peak and cool-down pulse rate check. This lesson is repeated (32). Keep data records throughout the year. Encourage students to check their goals and make sure they are realistic. Goals may need to be revised if they are unrealistic. Students can keep the score sheet in their portfolios.

Handout 6.2   Fitness Challenge Score Sheet

Name_____

Date 1_____

Date 2_____

	Exercise	Score	Goal	Score	Improvement
1.	_____	_____	_____	_____	_____
2.	_____	_____	_____	_____	_____
3.	_____	_____	_____	_____	_____
4.	_____	_____	_____	_____	_____
5.	_____	_____	_____	_____	_____
6.	_____	_____	_____	_____	_____

Lesson 29

Change the Game

Goals

- To improve cardiovascular endurance
- To improve coordination skills

Key Concepts

Sports can be modified to include more movement and less standing. Reducing the number of players on each team makes a more active game and increases participation and contact with the equipment. Small teams guarantee all students are involved.

Materials

1. Soccer balls or basketballs (one for every four students)
2. Cones (for soccer boundaries and goals)
3. Pinnies

Warm-Up: 5 Minutes

Select stretching and warm-up activities.

Activity: Change the Game

- Select either soccer or basketball and play a 2 versus 2 game instead of an 11 versus 11 or 5 versus 5 game.

- If you select soccer, play 2 versus 2 on small fields using cones for lines and for goals.
- Set up fields 30 × 25 yards with goals three yards wide.
- If you select basketball, play 2 versus 2 at each hoop.

Activity: Partner Run

Increase the running interval to six minutes. Refer to lesson 24 for specific instructions.

Cool-Down: 5 Mintues

Select stretching and cool-down activities.

Teaching Tips

Point out that opportunities to rest are not as great in a 2 versus 2 game compared to a regulation full-sized game. The opportunity to touch the ball more often is present. Ask children to review other games they play and consider how those games can be adjusted to promote involvement, participation, and activity.

Lesson 30

Rate Your Plate

Goals

- To compare the cholesterol, fat, and sodium contents from a variety of fast-food restaurant meals
- To design a lunch menu that follows the recommendations for heart-healthy eating based on selections from fast-food restaurants

Key Concepts

In our fast-paced society, it is often difficult to follow nutritional guidelines and consume heart-healthy meals. We are sometimes faced with the decision of eating at fast-food restaurants or not eating at all. There are often healthy choices available at these restaurants. The reason for discouraging frequent dining at fast-food restaurants is that many of these foods are high in sodium and fat. The recommendations for heart-healthy eating suggest a daily intake of no more than 300 milligrams of cholesterol, low fat content (on a 2,500 calorie intake not more than 70 grams of fat should be ingested, which reflects less than 30 percent of the calories from fat; of this, not more than one third should come from saturated fat), and not more than 3 grams of sodium per day.

Materials

1. Menus and comparisons of the nutrient content from at least three fast-food restaurants such as McDonald's, Taco Bell, Wendy's, and Burger King
2. Handout 6.3 Rate Your Plate (one per group)
3. Handout 6.4 Week 6, Family Activity: Mighty Mini Pizzas (one per student)

Activity: Rate Your Plate

- Group students in pairs. Hand out the menus and comparison sheets. Each pair should create a lunch menu from each of the fast-food restaurants and calculate the cholesterol, total fat, and sodium contents of the meals they picked.
- Have the students rate which of the meals followed the recommendations, or design a menu that would be healthier.

Teaching Tips

Students could rate three or four days from the school menu or sack lunches brought to school. For lesson 40, collect empty cereal boxes and nutrition analysis guides (USDA handbooks or cookbooks).

Handout 6.3   Rate Your Plate

Name_____

	Restaurant and food	Food group	Cholesterol (mg)	Total fat (gm)	Sodium (mg)
1.	_____	_____	_____	_____	_____
2.	_____	_____	_____	_____	_____
3.	_____	_____	_____	_____	_____
4.	_____	_____	_____	_____	_____

Design a heart-healthy lunch menu from fast-food restaurants.

Handout 6.4   Week 6, Family Activity: Mighty Mini Pizzas

Mighty mini pizzas are a great after-school snack. They provide carbohydrates for energy and are not hard to make. Try the following recipe:

Ingredients

Sourdough or plain English muffins, 1/2 for each pizza
Spaghetti sauce, 1 T. for each pizza
Mozzarella cheese, 1 T. for each pizza

Optional ingredients

Unsweetened pineapple chunks, green pepper slices, sliced mushrooms, chopped onions, sliced tomatoes

Directions

1. Halve the muffins.
2. Spread each half with the 1 T. of sauce.
3. Sprinkle with any or all of the optional ingredients you like.
4. Top each with 1 T. of cheese.
5. Place on cookie sheet and broil until cheese is bubbly.

Write a paragraph comparing the mini pizzas to the pizzas you usually eat.

Time: 20 minutes

Please return by _____.

CHAPTER 7

Week 7: Flexibility Fitness

Lessons 32, 33, and 34 include a special segment called Flex Focus. It emphasizes specific body parts in the warm-up for flexibility training. The purpose of this segment is to teach stretching exercises to improve flexibility for specific joints in the body.

WEEK 7

Lesson 31

Flex Moves

Goals

- To understand the meaning and importance of flexibility
- To introduce new vocabulary related to flexibility
- To teach students that some traditional stretching exercises can be harmful

Key Concepts

Flexibility is an important, but often overlooked part of health-related physical fitness. Flexibility can be improved through stretching exercises. Adequate flexibility permits freedom of movement and may prevent some types of injuries. Flexibility is the range of movement of a specific joint and its muscle groups. For example, at the shoulder the arm can move up and down, forward and back, and rotate in a circular motion. Have students stand up in enough space to move arms freely and demonstrate range of motion. The flexibility of a joint depends on the elasticity of muscles around the joint. Flexibility exercises should not be competitive. More flexibility is not always better because joints can be too loose and unstable.

Materials

1. Tape measure (for each pair)
2. Masking tape
3. Mats
4. Handout 7.1 Student Flexibility Profile (one per student)
5. Handout 7.2 Week 7, Family Activity: Cable Calisthenics (one per student)

Activity: Flex Moves

Organize your class into pairs and have them complete the four flexibility activities: sit and reach, back raises, V splits, and bridge up. Students record their results on handout 7.1 Student Flexibility Profile. After testing use the results to lead into discussion of flexibility. The following issues are important to mention:

1. There are no ideal standards for flexibility. Some children are more flexible than others. A child who can reach one inch past her toes is not less fit than a child who can reach five inches past his toes. However, too little flexibility means that joints cannot move easily and too much flexibility causes loose joints that may lead to dislocation.
2. To keep joints flexible, regular range of motion (ROM) exercises are essential. Flexible joints help prevent injuries. Ask students to describe other stretching activities to improve flexibility of specific body joints.
3. Show children the preferred stretches and the nonpreferred stretches and explain why the preferred stretch prevents injury (see fig. 7.1).
4. Describe the following for successful stretching practice:
   - Exhale when moving into stretch.
   - Breathe normally while holding stretch.
   - Inhale when releasing.
   - Always stretch slowly and never stretch by bobbing, bouncing, or jerking.

Preferred	Instead of
A. Lateral straddle stretch	Hurdler stretch

Reason—the knee is not placed in an unnatural position. It does not stress the cartilage in the knee.

B. One leg stretcher	The plough

Reason—does not promote forward head and hump back.

C. Sitting toe touch	Standing toe touch

Reason—reduces stress on the muscles of the back.

D. Knee to chest	Double leg lifts

Reason—reduces strain on the lower back.

Teaching Tips

For safe and beneficial stretching, hold a sustained stretch for three to five seconds. Slow and gentle

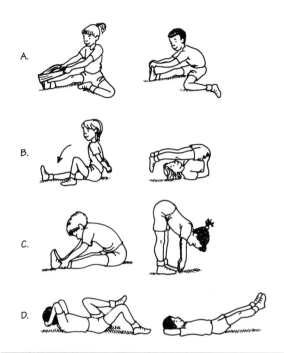

Fig. 7.1. Preferred and nonpreferred stretches

stretching helps reduce muscle tension. Bouncing movements produce a muscle contraction or tension in the muscle. Perform each stretch three times with relaxation between each stretch. Invite a speaker, such as an athletic trainer, physical therapist, aerobics instructor, dance instructor, or gymnastics coach to talk about stretching. Explain Cable Calisthenics worksheet (handout 7.2) and send home with children.

Play a Native American game, hacky sack. Use a regular hacky sack or a leather glove turned inside out. Players kick the object into the air and pass it around using only their feet. The object of the game is to see how long the object can stay in motion. This is an excellent activity for hip flexibility.

Handout 7.1   Student Flexibility Profile

Name_____

Date_____

1. Sit and reach (low-back stretch)
   Secure a tape measure on the floor or mat with masking tape. Sit on the floor with heels five to eight inches apart. Place the 15-inch mark at the heels with zero end toward the body. With one hand on top of the other and fingertips together, reach down and place hands on tape. Reach and hold for five seconds. Measure distance on measuring tape.

   Score_____

2. Back raises
   Lie on your tummy and lift head. Keep hands by side of body. Measure distance from the nose to the floor.

   Score_____

3. V splits
   Sit with feet apart in a V position. Measure distance between feet from heel to heel. Keep back of knees on ground.

   Score_____

4. Bridge up (no measurement)
   Lie on back with hands above the head, push up with hands and feet to make a bridge. Push stomach upward to the ceiling forming an upside down U with the body.

   Able to complete _____

   Unable to complete _____

Handout 7.2   Week 7, Family Activity: Cable Calisthenics

All children will spend some time watching TV, some a lot more than others. Two opportunities exist to exercise while watching TV. During programs, children can stretch. Using the warm-up and cool-down stretches, children can teach family members how to perform the stretch before the program begins, and let family members complete the stretch while watching TV.

In addition, during commercial breaks there is time to complete a more vigorous exercise, such as push-ups, sit-ups, or jumping jacks.

Use this worksheet to help children prepare a plan to help their family members exercise while watching TV.

Write the name of the three stretches and three exercises you would like your family to learn.

Stretches	Exercises
1.	1.
2.	2.
3.	3.

Pick three programs that you usually watch each week and who you will complete the stretches and exercises with.

Program	Family member
1.	1.
2.	2.
3.	3.

Directions

Get together a few minutes before the program begins to let the family members know what is going to happen. Ask the family members to carry out a stretch in each segment of the show and complete five repetitions of the selected exercise in each commercial break.

Complete the following:

1. How did the family members like the approach?

2. Did family members provide excuses about why they did not want to participate? If so, what were they?

Time: 30 minutes

Please return by _____.

WEEK 7

Lesson 32

Fitness Challenge II

Goals

- To improve lower-back flexibility
- To challenge students to meet their personal goals in specific exercises

Key Concepts

The primary causes of lower-back pain are inactivity and tension. Exercise can assist in preventing and reducing low-back pain. Prevention involves strengthening the abdominal muscles and increasing low-back flexibility.

Materials

1. Handout 6.2 Fitness Challenge Score Sheet from lesson 28
2. Mats

Warm-Up: 5 Minutes

Select stretching and warm-up activities. Give special emphasis to the low back and chest (see fig. 7.2). Lessons 32, 33, and 34 include a segment called Flex Focus. Different body joints and parts are selected and specific stretching exercises are introduced for that joint or part of the body.

Flex Focus: Chest (see fig. 7.2)

1. *Chest stretcher*
   In a prone (lying on stomach) position, lift upper body off the ground so the arms are straight. Complete five times.

2. *Swimmer*
   Tilt the trunk slightly forward. Imitate a freestyle swim stroke. Complete 10 to 12 strokes with each arm.

Flex Focus: Lower Back (see fig. 7.2)

1. *Sit and reach*
   Sit with knees slightly bent and feet pointed upward. Reach toward the toes. Bend forward from the hips. Try to pull the chin toward the knees. Hold for 10 to 20 seconds. Repeat two or three times.

2. *Back stretcher*
   Pull the right leg toward the chest by holding onto the hamstrings. Keep the left leg slightly bent. Hold for 20 to 30 seconds. Switch legs. Repeat two or three times.

3. *Pill bug*
   Pull both legs to the chest by holding onto the hamstrings. Curl the head up toward the knees. Hold for 5 to 15 seconds. Relax. Repeat two or three times.

Activity: Fitness Challenge II

- Use the directions from lesson 28.
- Children repeat the original challenge and try to improve their score on each exercise.
- Ask children to set new goals. Spend time discussing goal setting.
- Explain that some children will score higher than others and this is to be expected because some children are naturally more talented than others.
- Emphasize that everyone can improve. The focus should be physical fitness and improvement rather than comparison to other children.

Cool-Down: 5 Minutes

Select stretching and cool-down activities.

Teaching Tips

Spend a few minutes during cool-down phase asking students to evaluate their goal setting based on their performance in this lesson.

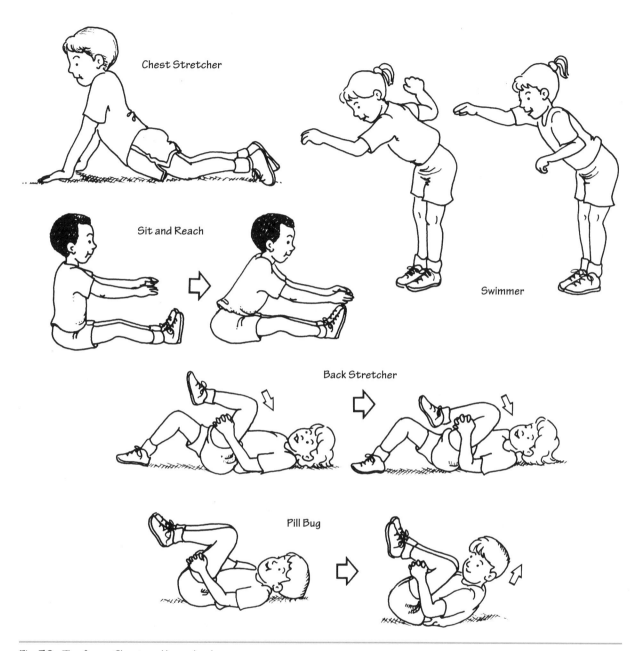

Fig. 7.2. Flex focus: Chest and lower back

Lesson 33

Soccer Knockdown

Goals

- To develop upper and lower leg flexibility
- To improve cardiovascular endurance
- To improve soccer skills

Key Concepts

This version of soccer provides ample opportunity for successful experiences with players on small teams. Teams with fewer players increase scoring opportunities and contact time with the soccer ball.

Materials

1. Twenty cones
2. Six soccer balls

Warm-Up: 5 Minutes

Select stretching and warm-up activities. Give special emphasis to the legs (see fig. 7.3).

Flex Focus: Upper Legs (see fig. 7.3)

1. *Sitting stretcher*
   Sit with soles of feet together, legs flat on the floor. Place hands on knees and lean forearms against knees; resist while trying to raise knees. Hold five to seven seconds, then relax.

2. *Hip and thigh stretcher*
   Place right knee directly above right ankle and stretch left leg backward so the knee touches the floor. If necessary, place hands on floor for balance. Press pelvis forward and downward and hold. Repeat on other side.

Flex Focus: Lower Legs (see fig. 7.3)

1. *Calf stretch*
   Stand with right leg forward and left leg back. Keep left leg straight and bend right leg. Lean forward, keeping heel of left foot on ground. Hold for three seconds. Repeat for right leg.

2. *Shin stretcher*
   Kneel on both knees, turn to right, press down on right ankle with right hand, and hold. Keep hips thrust forward to avoid hyperflexing knees. Do not sit on heels. Repeat on left side.

Activity: Soccer Knockdown

- Divide class into four teams to play two separate games of Soccer Knockdown.
- For each game, set up two lines of cones, 30 to 40 yards apart (see fig. 7.4).
- Four cones are spaced five or six yards apart.
- The objective is to knock down the opposing team's cones with the ball by dribbling or passing.
- Start with one ball per game, then introduce a second and third ball.
- The player who knocks down a cone has to pick it up, leave the ball where it is, and run back to his or her own line of cones before rejoining the game.
- Play four periods of four minutes each. Players keep track of their own score.

Cool-Down: 5 Minutes

Select stretching and cool-down activities.

Teaching Tips

Players must play the ball and not push, shove, or kick opposing players. For any of these offenses penalize by subtracting a point from the offending players. Emphasize cooperative team play. If players are defending a cone, they must remain at least three yards from cone.

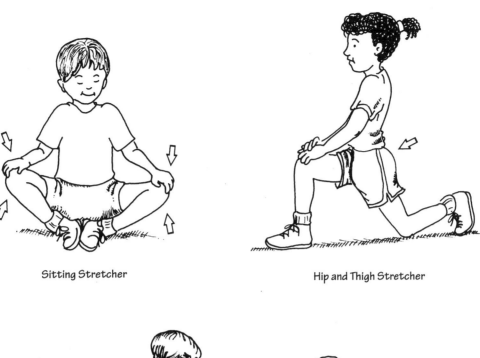

Sitting Stretcher

Hip and Thigh Stretcher

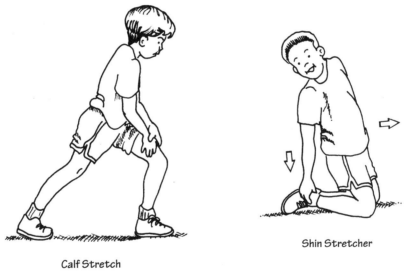

Calf Stretch

Shin Stretcher

Fig. 7.3. Flex focus: Legs

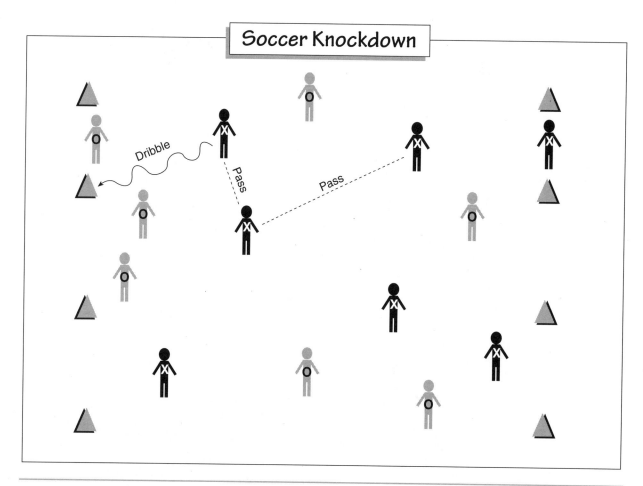

Fig. 7.4. Soccer knockdown

WEEK 7

Lesson 34

Aerobic Kickball

Goals

- To improve cardiovascular endurance
- To improve neck and shoulder flexibility
- To improve basic ball skills

Key Concepts

Take great care stretching neck muscles. Constantly and vigorously rotating the head is not advisable. Use slow movements and hold stretch for three seconds.

Materials

1. Cones for bases
2. One playground ball

Warm-Up: 5 Minutes

Select stretching and warm-up activities. Give special emphasis to shoulder and neck flexibility in the warm-up (see fig. 7.5).

Flex Focus: Neck (see fig. 7.5)

1. *Neck stretch*
   Keeping shoulders back and spine straight, slowly roll the head to the left shoulder, straighten, then roll toward right shoulder, straighten. Repeat five times. Do not roll the head in a fast, circular manner or roll head backward.

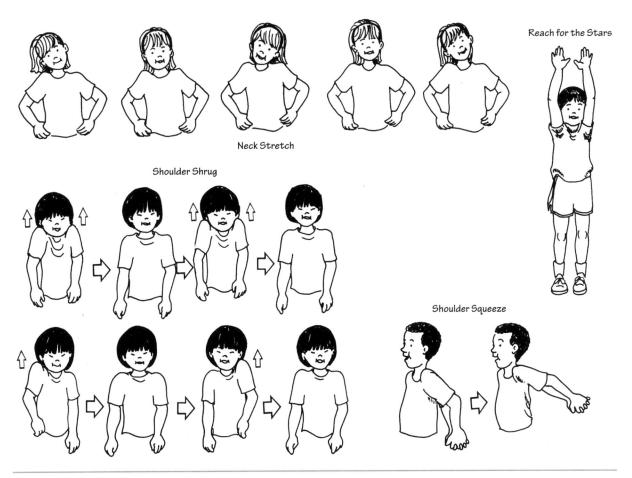

Fig. 7.5. Flex focus: Shoulder and neck

Flex Focus: Shoulder (see fig. 7.5)

1. ***Shoulder shrug (helps to reduce muscle tension in neck and shoulders)***
   Shrug both shoulders up toward your ears. Hold and repeat. Shrug shoulders forward as far as possible. Hold and repeat. Shrug shoulders backward as far as possible. Hold and repeat. Shrug each shoulder opposite ways, up and down. Hold and repeat.

2. ***Reach for the stars***
   Hold both hands together and reach above the head.

3. ***Shoulder squeeze (stretches back of arms and shoulders)***
   Hold both hands behind your back (standing position). Keeping legs straight, bend forward at waist. Raise arms up over head from behind (repeat two or three times).

Activity: Aerobic Kickball

- Divide the class into two teams.
- The batting team is then divided into three groups, A, B, and C.
- The fielding team spreads out in the field.
- One member of batting group A is up to bat and kicks a stationary ball into the field. All of batting group A run around the bases (no passing).
- The fielder collects the ball and runs to the pitching mound.
- Everyone else on the fielding team runs to line up behind the player with the ball, and the ball is passed back over the heads of the fielding team.
- The batting group A has to reach home plate before the ball reaches the back person on the fielding team.

- A member of each batting group (groups switch after three kicks) has a turn, then the fielding and batting teams switch places.
- Batting team has the right of way.

Cool-Down: 5 Minutes

Select stretching and cool-down activities.

Teaching Tips

If students are used to traditional kickball, they may question this new version. Emphasize that in traditional kickball there is a lot of standing around. This new game provides more activity and involvement. Encourage cooperative and supportive behaviors. You can vary the activities of the fielders (students can form a circle around the pitcher's mound and pass ball around circle). You can adjust the distance between the bases.

Lesson 35

The Label Fable

WEEK 7

Goals

- To reinforce the importance of understanding nutritional information on labels
- To distinguish heart-healthy products

Key Concepts

Previous lessons have emphasized the importance of consuming heart-healthy foods. Most of these include fresh, nonprocessed foods. How then, do packaged foods fit into planning nutritious, low-fat, low-cholesterol meals? The key is learning to decipher package labels when choosing what to buy. The ability to distinguish between heart-healthy products and those laden with unwanted fats depends on your mastery of label vocabulary.

Materials

1. Handout 7.3 Reader's Theater "The Label Fable" (10 copies)
2. Empty cracker boxes

Activity: The Label Fable

- Select 10 volunteers for roles in the reader theater.
- Provide each reader with a copy of "The Label Fable."
- Have available at least two empty boxes of crackers to use for props.
- Perform the Readers' Theater and discuss with the class the importance of not being deceived by fancy labels.
- Working in groups, the students can create their own Readers' Theater or a cartoon strip that illustrates the concepts developed in "The Label Fable."

Note: This lesson reprinted with permission from the July/August issue of *Learning91*, copyright © 1991, Springhouse Corporation, 1111 Bethlehem Pike, Springhouse PA 19477. All rights reserved.

Teaching Tip

Highlight each character part in script.

Handout 7.3   Readers' Theater "The Label Fable"

Characters:

Teacher	Narrator 2
Student 1	Wes
Student 2	Ryan
Student 3	Cracker 1
Narrator 1	Cracker 2

Teacher: Our back-to-school picnic is Friday afternoon.

Student 1: What food are we going to have?

Student 2: Hot dogs and sodas?

Student 3: I can bring *Crinkle Crunchers*.

Teacher: Whoa! We've been studying about heart-healthy foods.

Student 2: And healthy snacks.

Student 1: Why don't we help our own hearts?

Teacher: Right. These aren't just lessons for school. You can use them everywhere.

Student 3: Let's form a committee and plan a super picnic.

Student 1: Let's see. How about fruit juice and bananas and. . .

Narrator 1: The class spent the next hour planning for the picnic. They put together a menu that included foods from all our food groups. Students volunteered to buy apple juice, raisins, vegetables, dip, and other things.

Narrator 2: Wes and Ryan offered to buy crackers for the dip. At the store, they stood staring at all the cracker boxes.

Wes: We're supposed to pick a cracker that's heart healthy.

Ryan: How about *Wheat Wonders*? Wheat's healthy.

Wes: Or this one—*Nutritious Nibbles*. It sounds healthy.

Cracker 1: You're right, kid. *Nutritious Nibbles* is your best bet. Look, I'm shaped like animals—kids love animals.

Cracker 2: You think you're the best? You're full of fat and low in fiber. They won't pick you. They want *Wheat Wonders*. I'm low in fat and loaded with wheat fiber.

Cracker 1: But you're boring. Kids don't care what's good for them. They'll pick me. I've got style.

Narrator 1: As the crackers argue about who's best, Wes and Ryan try to remember what they learned in class.

Wes: They should be low in fat, especially saturated fat like butter.

Ryan: Yeah, and low in cholesterol.

Wes: Look! This one says "No Cholesterol" right on the front.

Ryan: Wes, that's just an advertising gimmick.

Narrator 2: The boys know that crackers are made from flour, flour comes from plants, and plants have no cholesterol.

Wes: You're right. Well, let's make sure there's no saturated fat. Let's check the ingredients for butter and oil.

Ryan: Nope, no butter. There's oil, though. Is safflower oil good or bad?

Narrator 1: In class the boys learned that safflower oil—like most oils—is made mostly of polyunsaturated fats.

Wes: It's a good oil. Coconut oil and palm oil are the only bad ones, remember? So let's buy this one.

Ryan: Wait. Besides the kind of fat, we need to make sure it's low in fat. The label says four grams of fat per serving, and a serving's only five crackers. That seems like a lot of fat.

Wes: Look at these. They have only two grams of fat for five crackers. We'd better take these instead.

Cracker 1: Rats! They chose *Heart Smart* crackers instead of us.

Narrator 2: Wes and Ryan used the information they learned in class to read the package labels and choose the best cracker.

CHAPTER 8

Week 8: Strength Fitness

Lessons 37, 38, and 39 include a special segment called Muscle Moment. It emphasizes specific body parts in the warm-up for strength training. The purpose of this segment is to teach exercises to increase strength of specific areas of the body.

Lesson 36

Muscle Search

WEEK 8

Goals

- To learn the names and locations of muscle groups
- To learn the actions of specific muscle groups

Key Concepts

Muscular strength and endurance are fitness components that relate to cardiovascular health. An effective muscular system allows the body to participate in vigorous activities. Learning the names and actions of muscles provides an essential knowledge base for developing exercise routines.

Materials

1. Muscle fig. 8.1 (one per each pair)
2. Masking tape
3. Felt-tip pens
4. Blank paper for drawing outline

Activity: Muscle Search

Use fig. 8.1 to help children locate the major muscle groups. Divide class by gender into pairs and provide each pair with masking tape and a pen. Using pieces of masking tape, help children tape the name of the major muscle groups on each other. Place tape on exterior garments. Write names on tape first before placing on body. Use the muscle action chart to help children determine the action of each major muscle.

Muscle Action Chart*

	Muscle	Action
1.	Biceps	Bends elbow
2.	Triceps	Straightens elbow
3.	Deltoid	Lifts arm and shoulder
4.	Quadriceps	Straightens knee
5.	Hamstrings	Bends knee
6.	Rectus abdominis	Bends hip and waist
7.	Latissimus dorsi	Pulls up body
8.	Trapezius	Lifts shoulders
9.	Pectoralis	Pushing, hugging
10.	Calves	Bends ankle

* Represents the most basic muscle movement.

Teaching Tips

Students may be sensitive to others placing tape on certain parts of their body. Give students the option of placing their own piece of tape on the muscle. When students have finished labeling their own body, have them make two body outlines (front and back). Transfer knowledge of muscles by writing names on outlines. Place outlines in student portfolios. Make students aware that most muscles are bilateral (on both sides of body).

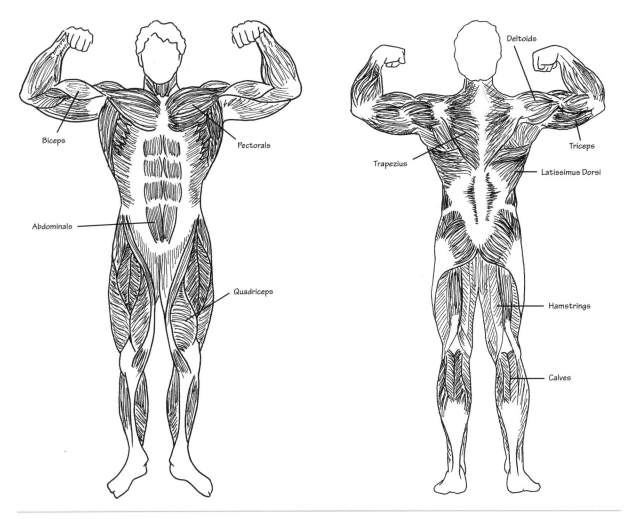

Fig. 8.1. The muscular system

WEEK 8

Lesson 37

Parachute Power

Goals

- To improve arm, shoulder, and abdominal strength and endurance
- To improve cardiovascular endurance

Key Concepts

Children often lack upper body strength. Arm and shoulder strength are required for most lifting and carrying activities. Give regular emphasis to improving upper body fitness.

Materials

1. Parachute
2. Eight to 10 foam or rubber balls

Warm-Up: 5 Minutes

Select stretching and warm-up activities. The Muscle Moment features a specific body part and provides exercises to strengthen that part. Give special emphasis to the arms, shoulders, and chest.

Muscle Moment: Arms and Shoulders

The triceps muscle is on the back of the upper arm. The push-up uses the triceps muscle to help lift you off the floor. The biceps muscle is on the front of the upper arm and allows you to curl your arm and bend your elbow. As you eat food, the biceps muscle allows you to move the fork to your mouth. The deltoid muscle helps lift objects and is used in throwing. Complete five repetitions of each of the following (see chapter 13 for diagrams) to strengthen these three muscles.

1. *Side standers*
   Lie in prone position with chest touching floor, legs and feet together. Hands are directly under shoulders. Raise body in push-up fashion. At full arm extension, rotate body one quarter turn to left, supporting weight on right hand and foot. Return to starting position. Rotate body to the right, supporting weight on left hand and foot. Return to starting position.
2. *Crab legs*
   Support weight on hands and feet. Alternatively, kick legs out and away from body—this is one repetition.
3. *Crab walker*
   From sitting position, push body off ground and support weight on hands and feet. Move body forward and backward three steps—this is one repetition.

Muscle Moment: Chest

The main chest muscles are the pectorals. The pectorals are shaped like a fan and help to cover and protect the upper ribs. The pectorals help you pull the arm across the front of the body. They are used in hugging. Complete five repetitions of each of the following to strengthen the pectorals.

1. *Push-ups or modified push-ups*
   Lie on stomach with chest touching the floor and feet together. Hands are under the shoulders. Push and raise body by extending arms. Raise body in straight line, not allowing back to sway. Lower body until chin touches ground.

2. *Chest strength*
   Lie on bench or floor and do "flys" with weights (use canned food, books).

Activity: Parachute Power

1. Tidal waves
   Students grip parachute near outer edge with hands, palm down, and shake vigorously! Vary size of waves.
2. Chute scoot
   Grasp chute in right hand, move clockwise and vary movements with skip, jog, run, hop. Switch hands and change direction.
3. Popcorn
   Place foam or rubber balls on chute. Shake until all balls are bounced off the chute.
4. Keep on rollin'
   Hold chute waist high, roll it forward, then move backward unrolling the chute.
5. Parapull
   All students pull chute at same time, leaning back and holding for 10 seconds.
6. Strength stretcher
   Students grasp chute and face outward while holding chute overhead. On signal, students pull and hold for 10 seconds.
7. Cannonball
   Place ball in center of chute and lift up and vigorously down to shoot ball toward ceiling.
8. Sit-ups
   Sit down with legs underneath the parachute, while grasping the chute with overhand grip. On signal, all students complete a sit-up. Repeat 15 times.

Cool-Down: 5 Minutes

Select stretching and cool-down activities.

Teaching Tips

Use cues, such as one whistle means go to the left. Chute Scoot should last 5 to 10 minutes. In Popcorn, designate a ball chaser.

WEEK 8

Lesson 38
Partner Challenge

Goals

- To improve abdominal and lower-back strength
- To improve cardiovascular endurance

Key Concepts

Back pain can be a result of inactivity and lack of back and abdominal strength. For this reason, it is essential that children as well as adults learn and practice exercises that strengthen the back.

Materials

1. Ball (one per pair)
2. Jump rope (one per pair)

Warm-Up: 5 Minutes

Select stretching and warm-up activities. Give special emphasis to the abdominals and lower back.

Muscle Moment: Abdominals

The rectus abdominus or the abdominals support and protect body organs. The abdominals allow you to move your spine. Demonstrate four exercises that strengthen the abdominal muscles. Encourage children to start with five repetitions of each exercise.

1. *Crunches*
   Lie on back with legs together and knees bent, forming a 90-degree angle. Hands are behind head. Bring knees and elbows together, directly over waist area. Return to starting position.
2. *Bridge back*
   Begin on hands and knees in crawling position with feet shoulder-width apart. Tighten abdominal muscles and arch back as high as possible. Return to starting position. Emphasize importance of tightening abdominal muscles (students should feel it).
3. *Reverse sit-ups (works lower portion of abdomen)*
   Lie on back with bent legs together and arms and hands extended over head. Bend at the

waist bringing knees as close to chest as possible. Return to starting position.
4. *Obliques (strengthens side of torso)*
   Lie on back, knees bent, feet on floor, with hands held lightly behind head. Lift one shoulder and upper torso off floor, twisting toward opposite knee. Do not pull head and neck with hands. Return to starting position and repeat other side. Press spine to floor so hips do not roll.

Muscle Moment: Lower Back

The latissimus dorsi (shortened to lats) are triangle shaped and extend from under the shoulders to the lower back. Lift your right arm over your head and place your left hand under your right shoulder. Slowly pull your right elbow to your right hip and feel your lats muscle contract. The lats help you climb a rope. The trapezius is located on the upper back below the neck and lifts the shoulders up and down as in a shoulder shrug.

1. *Curl-ups*
   In this exercise the lower back acts as a stabilizer. Lie on floor with hands on upper thighs, reach up until back comes off the ground.
2. *Chest raises*
   In this activity the lower back is a prime mover. Lie on stomach with arms at side and raise chest and head from the ground.

Activity: Partner Challenge

- Pair up students. Pairs face each other on opposite sides of an area with a centerline between them.
- Partners jog to meet in the middle and take turns challenging each other with an exercise. Partners jog to the outside to complete their challenges.
- Provide a 30-second period, then students meet in the middle and tell the other how many times they completed the exercise.
- Then select new exercises.

Cool-Down: 5 Minutes

Select stretching and cool-down activities.

Teaching Tips

Change partners periodically. Teacher can challenge class with a number of repetitions or a specific activity. Use additional exercises in chapter 13. You can use ball skill and jump rope challenges.

WEEK 8

Lesson 39
Super Circuit

Goals

- To perform a variety of strength skills in station format
- To improve leg strength

Key Concepts

Muscular strength is the ability to lift or move an object. It is defined as the ability to complete one repetition of a specific exercise. Use the example of Olympic weightlifting, lifting a maximum weight once.

Muscular endurance is the ability to repeatedly move your body or an object. Use the example of the number of sit-ups performed in one minute, or completing many repetitions of lifting a certain amount of weight.

Materials

1. Tape player
2. Station cards with names of exercises
3. Cones

Warm-Up: 5 Minutes

Select stretching and warm-up activities. Give special emphasis to the legs.

Muscle Moment: Upper Legs

The hamstrings are the muscles on the back of the top part of your leg. The hamstrings allow you to bend the knee. All running activities will use the hamstring muscles. The thigh muscles are one of the strongest muscle groups in the body. The quadriceps are on the front part of the upper leg. Quad means four and there are four long muscles that start near the hip and extend down to the knee. The quadriceps help you straighten your leg.

The following exercises use the quadriceps and hamstring muscle groups (in addition to others).

Demonstrate the exercises designed to strengthen the upper legs.

1. *Stride jumps*
   Stand with feet together and hands on hips. Hop off the ground so feet are spread to sides about three feet apart. Return to starting position. Similar to jumping jacks with no arm movements. Complete 15 repetitions.
2. *Leg extensions*
   Kneel on floor and place hands in front of body. Extend leg behind body and lift. Switch legs. Complete 10 repetitions with each leg.

Muscle Moment: Lower Leg

The calf muscle (gastrocnemius) lifts the foot up and down and is used to stand on the toes and balance. The following exercises use the lower leg.

1. *Heel lifts*
   Lift heels off the ground, bend at the knee slightly, and push off toes into an upright position. Knees should not go past a 90-degree angle. Complete 10 repetitions.
2. *Ten jumps higher*
   Make a series of 10 jumps, each one higher than the previous one. Complete three repetitions.
3. *Sprint starts*
   Begin on all fours with right knee forward. On command "set" students raise knees off the ground. On command "go," students run for 10 yards. Complete three repetitions.

Activity: Super Circuit

Using the following strength exercises establish stations for each exercise. Divide students into groups of three. Students exercise for 30 seconds at each station, jog around the outside of the stations for 30 seconds, then rotate to the next station. The exercise and run format continues until students have completed one circuit. Provide a rest, then repeat.

1. Bridge backs
2. Stride jumps
3. Jack-in-the box
4. Crab legs
5. Crab walkers
6. Chest raises
7. Crunches
8. Side standers
9. Curl-ups
10. Jump twisters

Cool-Down: 5-Minutes

Select stretching and cool-down activities.

Teaching Tips

You can vary the length of the exercise and jog segments according to fitness levels. Include a walk rather than a jog if necessary.

WEEK 8

Lesson 40

The Case of the Label Connection

Goals

- To investigate cereal box labels for evidence of heart-healthy or heart-hazardous ingredients
- To make informed consumer choices when selecting breakfast cereals
- To determine "hidden" fat in breakfast cereals

Key Concepts

Students should understand the coding of package labels to make better selections. The new USDA label requirements include a more complete format with information listed as percentages.

Materials

1. Figure 8.2 The Case of the Label Connection (one per group)
2. Empty cereal boxes (at least two or three per group)

3. Handout 8.1 Week 8, Family Activity: Fixer Upper (one per student)

Activity: The Case of the Label Connection

- Instruct each student to complete the Case of the Label Connection worksheet. Discuss with the students which cereals they would pick and why.
- Organize the students into groups and instruct each group to compare the results of their worksheets and discuss their results. Next, examine the contents and labels of at least two cereals.
- Compare these cereals with the Krispies brand and write a paragraph discussing their findings. Numerically rank the cereals.

The Case of the LABEL CONNECTION

Inspector Smart is investigating Krispies cereal for heart-hazardous ingredients. Study the label below and help him find the evidence. Then investigate two other cereal labels and compare.
Which cereal is heart -healthiest?

Krispies

Nutrition Information Per Serving

Serving size .... 1 cup
Servings per container 12
Calories 90
Protein .... 3 grams
Carbohydrate .... 22 grams
Fat 1gram
Sodium .... 190 milligrams

Percentage of U.S. Recommended Daily Allowances (U.S. RDA)

Protein 4%	Vitamin D 10%
Vitamin A 25%	Vitamin B6 .... 25%
Vitamin C .... •	Folic Acid 25%
Thiamine (B) 25%	Vitamin B12 ..... 25%
Riboflavin (B2) 25%	Phosphorous ... 25%
Niacin 5%	Magnesium 10%
Calcium .... •	Zinc 10%
Iron 25%	Copper 25%

*Contains less than 2% of the U.S. RDA of these nutrients

Ingredients: Whole Wheat, Wheat Bran, Sugar, Raisins, Dried Apples (with Sulfur Dioxide, a Preservative), Almonds, Natural Flavoring, Salt, Corn Syrup, Coconut Oil, and Artificial Flavor. BHA added to preserve freshness.

1. First, check the nutrition information.
What's the serving size? _____
How many grams of fat are in each serving? _____

2. Next, check the ingredients list.
Do you find extra fat or oil? _____
If yes, name it. _____
Is it saturated, monosaturated, or polyunsaturated?
How do you know? _____

3. The first item in the ingredients list is the one that makes up most (at least 60%) of the product. There's less of the second item, even less of the third, and so on.
What's listed first? _____

4. Is the cereal cholesterol free?
Why, or why not? _____

5. Do you think Inspector Smart will find Krispies to be a heart-healthy cereal?_____
Why, or why not? _____
_____
_____
_____

	Krispies	Cereal B	Cereal C
Serving size			
Fat/serving			
Extra fat or oil?			
Type of fat			
1st ingredient			
Cholesterol-free?			
Heart-healthy?			

Fig. 8.2. The case of the label connection

Handout 8.1   Week 8, Family Activity: Fixer Upper

Find one of your family's favorite recipes and show how you can make it more heart healthy. Then try it and rate it on the form below. Use the suggestions from Handout 2.6 Week 2, Family Activity: Out With the Fat, In With the Lean on reducing fat, saturated fat, and cholesterol, and information from nutrition lessons, especially lesson 20, The Final Four Plus Two.

Recipe

How we changed it

Did you like it? Why or why not?

Time: 30 minutes
Please return by _____.

CHAPTER 9

Week 9: Healthy Lifestyle

The lessons explain the F.I.T. formula to help students plan their own fitness programs. Students plan a fitness program for themselves. The nutrition information describes a heart-healthy approach to cooking pizza.

WEEK 9

Lesson 41

Get F.I.T.

Goal

- To understand how much, how long, and how hard to exercise

Key Concepts

Technology has taken most people out of working in fields and factories and put them behind desks—and in front of computers. With more conveniences we are doing less and less manual work. Cars, elevators, escalators, garage door openers, food processors, drive-up windows, and remote controls have reduced physical activity for most people. To increase physical activity levels students should understand how to plan their own physical fitness regimes. F.I.T. stands for frequency, intensity, and time, which should be followed when planning aerobic exercise programs.

Materials

1. Handout 9.1 Weekly Exercise Planner (one for each student)
2. 12 × 18 inch drawing paper

Activity: Get F.I.T.

1. Introduce a prescription for aerobic exercise: F.I.T.
   Ask students the following questions:
   - F = Frequency. How many times a week should you exercise to be physically fit? (a minimum of three days per week)
   - I = Intensity. How hard should you exercise? (until you reach your target heart rate or approximately 150–170 beats per minute)
   - T = Time. How long should you exercise? (continuously for 20 minutes)
2. Ask students to describe the benefits of following F.I.T.
   - Body is able to use more oxygen.

- Heart grows stronger (won't have to beat as many times when resting).
- Improved blood circulation, which reduces the risk of heart disease.
- Strengthens muscles and bones.
- Helps you sleep better.
- Reduces stress.
- Increases your level of energy and concentration.
- Increases self confidence—you will feel better about yourself.

Use the weekly planner in handout 9.1 to help children determine how they will meet the F.I.T. guidelines.

Teaching Tips

Exercise includes household and gardening chores as well as sports and exercise. You can include these on the weekly planner. For an additional activity try the following. Divide your class into groups and ask them to list possible explanations for the following facts:

- People living in the United States are the world's most overweight.
- Today's kids are less fit than children growing up 10 years ago.

After the groups share their lists, split the class into two-person teams. Have each team fold a sheet of 12 × 18 inch drawing paper in half and label one side "1895" and the other side "1995". Challenge the teams to illustrate how life today has become less physically demanding by depicting various family members doing common tasks. For example, folks on the 1895 side could be shown splitting logs with an ax, hoeing a vegetable garden, and using a hand pump to get water. Those depicted on the 1995 side could be cutting wood with a chain saw, turning the soil with a Rototiller, and getting water from an outdoor spigot. After the teams share their illustrations, post the pictures on a bulletin board.

Handout 9.1   Weekly Exercise Planner

Activities

Monday _____

Tuesday _____

Wednesday _____

Thursday _____

Friday _____

Saturday _____

Sunday _____

Directions: Write in the name of your planned activity or exercise and how long you plan to exercise.

Follow-Up: After planning and then completing the exercise schedule, you can review the plans and determine how well you kept to the plan.

Answer the following:

Was it too ambitious?

What changes need to be made?

Were there obstacles that prevented you from completing your plan?

Lesson 42

Windows of Opportunity

Goals

- To improve cardiovascular endurance
- To improve muscular strength

Key Concepts

The F.I.T. guidelines suggested in lesson 41 provide sound prescriptions for staying fit. However, many individuals may not be able to meet those guidelines. If this is the case students should understand that some exercise is better than none. Accumulating five minutes of exercise at different times during the day will improve physical fitness.

Materials

1. Exercise cards
2. Whistle
3. Balls (one per pair) optional
4. Cones

Warm-Up: 5 minutes

Select stretching and warm-up activities.

Activity: Windows of Opportunity

- Set up an area 40 × 30 yards with cones.
- Divide class into pairs.

- One member of the pair is inside the playing area. The other partner is on the perimeter of the playing area.
- Students inside jog in the playing area in and out of cones (or polyspots) and pick out their partner on the outside to complete a high five on a whistle cue.
- After completing a high five, the outside player does 10 repetitions of an exercise (e.g., mountain climbers, jumping jacks, sit-ups). The players inside keep jogging.
- The activity continues with different tasks for the players to complete with a partner.
- Use cards to show the activity requested.
- After four minutes, change the players from the perimeter to the inside.
- Use balls to provide additional activities (e.g., players dribble a basketball and pass to an outside player, who throws it back to the inside player, who keeps dribbling).

Cool-Down: 5 Minutes

Select stretching and cool-down activities.

Teaching Tips

Use polyspots or cones as designated markers for children on the outside. When introducing balls, give specific instructions regarding the types of passes, such as bounce pass or chest pass. Provide teaching tips on each technique.

Lesson 43

Fitness Club

Goals

- To help children select motivating workout activities in completing their own workout
- To develop cardiovascular endurance

Key Concepts

A worthy goal of school physical education is to provide students the knowledge, skills, and abilities to plan their own exercise programs. An objective of this program is to help students create an active lifestyle. To achieve this objective students should be prepared to organize and plan their own physical activity program.

Materials

1. Music
2. Equipment based on student workouts
3. Student copies of club lessons

Warm-Up: 5 Minutes

Select stretching and warm-up activities (student designed).

Activity: Fitness Club

- Use the student-designed workouts or suggest activity options (e.g., jumping rope, 3 versus 3 basketball, 2 versus 2 volleyball, 3 versus 3 soccer, exercise stations with music).

- Other activities can be set up depending on facilities, equipment, and student interest.

Cool-Down: 5 Minutes

Select stretching and cool-down activities (student designed).

Teaching Tips

Provide flexibility in activity choices, but aim for continuous aerobic activity for 20 minutes. A juice bar may also be included (to reinforce the concept of "club"). Repeat this lesson once every three weeks to reinforce the club concept.

Club activities should be open to all students. Groups should not exclude any student and should emphasize participation and fun. Students can select their own music. It needs to be screened for appropriateness. The Fitness Club activities can be set up on a regular basis (once every three weeks) throughout the school year.

WEEK 9

Lesson 44

Cross-Country Kickball

Goal

- To improve cardiovascular endurance

Key Concepts

This version of kickball creates an opportunity for constant movement while keeping the familiar "kick and run" format. Give emphasis to activity and participation rather than winning and competition.

Materials

1. Bases
2. Four cones
3. One kickball

Warm-Up: 5 Minutes

Select stretching and warm-up activities.

Activity: Cross-Country Kickball

- Form two equal teams.
- Place a cone 15 to 20 yards behind each base (see fig. 9.1). Bases are placed 50 yards apart.
- The runner crosses first base, and continues on a cross-country run around the outside cones whether safe or out. The game continues.
- The goal is to complete the run before three outs. There may be a number of runners on the course at the same time and the defense may not tag them out.
- Outs are recorded by catching fly balls or being thrown out at first base.
- The kicking team's goal is to complete as many runs as possible before three outs.
- A run is scored if runner completes the course before three outs are made.
- Foul balls are outs, but kicker runs the course.

Cross Country Kickball

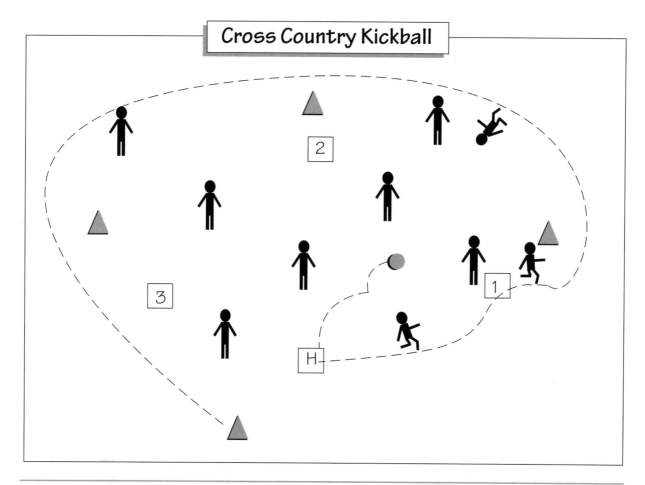

Fig. 9.1. Cross-country kickball

Cool-Down: 5 Minutes

Select stretching and cool-down activities.

Teaching Tips

A "one pitch per player" rule eliminates stalling by the kicking team (a badly pitched ball can be called and repitched). Teacher may want to pitch.

This activity was designed by physical education specialist Lefty Chell from Lassen View Elementary School, Chico, California.

WEEK 9

Lesson 45
Pizza Puzzler

Goals

- To review heart-healthy foods
- To design an individual heart-healthy pizza

Key Concepts

Everyday favorite foods, such as pizza, can be heart healthy by choosing low-fat, low-cholesterol alternatives. Pizza made with a high-quality flour, low-fat mozzarella cheese, and nutritious fat-free toppings can be a part of your heart-healthy lifestyle and be enjoyable too!

Materials

1. Fat Busters fig. 9.2 (one per group)
2. Pizza Puzzler pieces fig. 9.3 (one per group)
3. Handout 9.2 Week 9, Family Activity: Family Fitness Log (one per student)

Activity: Pizza Puzzler

- Randomly hand out one "piece" of the Pizza Puzzler to each student. Have them silently locate three other students with the piece that fits their puzzle. This is their cooperative and collaborative team.

- Instruct team members to answer the questions on each pizza piece.
- When all the questions have been answered, put the puzzle back together and design your own heart-healthy pizza.
- To conclude the lesson, each group should discuss their results with the class.

Teaching Tips

You can organize class members into groups of four.

Note: This lesson reprinted with permission from the July/August issue of *Learning91*, copyright © 1991, Springhouse Corporation, 1111 Bethlehem Pike, Springhouse, PA 19477. All rights reserved.

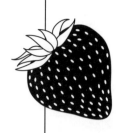

Fat Busters

Help your heart. Pick low-fat foods and fix them without adding fat. Discuss these tips as a family, then post them in your kitchen.They'll help you knock some fat and cholesterol out of your family meals.

Instead-ofs

Salad Dressing	Use lemon juice, fat-free dressing, or a bit of vegetable oil-based dressing.
Butter, shortening	Use liquid margarine or vegetable oil. In baking, try whole-grain flours to offset any flavor loss.
Mayonnaise, sour cream	Use buttermilk, plain nonfat yogurt, or blender-whipped low-fat cottage cheese.
Whole milk	Use skim or low-fat milk in pudding, soup, and baking.
Eggs	Use two whites for each whole egg in recipes for muffins, cookies, puddings, and pancakes. In scrambled eggs, use one whole egg per serving, extra whites for larger servings.

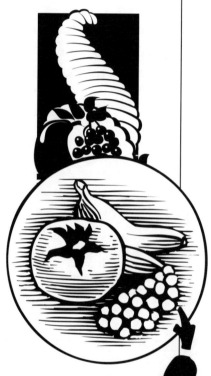

How-tos

Vegetables	Steam, boil, or bake, or stir-fry in a bit of vegetable oil. Season with lemon juice, herbs, and spices, not butter or sauce.
Meat, poultry, and fish	Choose lean cuts. Trim fat and poultry skin before eating. Simmer cuts, or roast, bake, or broil on a rack. Chill broth, soup, and stew until the fat solidifies; spoon off and discard. On a meatless day each week, eat whole grains and beans or other legumes for protein.
Pots and pans	Use nonstick cookware so extra fat is not necessary.

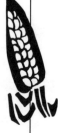

Fig. 9.2. Fat busters

Pizza Puzzler

Can a pizza be heart-healthy? To find out, "cut into" the pizza below and distribute the pieces to your teammates. After all the questions have been answered, put the puzzle back together, then use what you learned to design a heart-healthy pizza on the back.

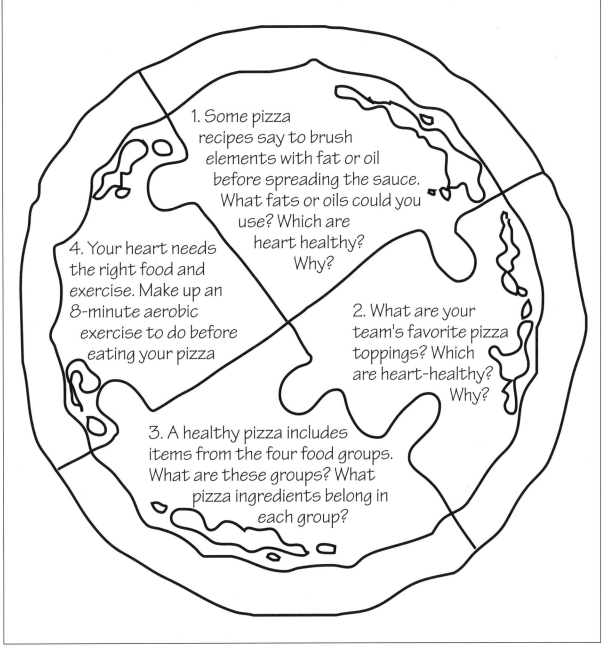

1. Some pizza recipes say to brush elements with fat or oil before spreading the sauce. What fats or oils could you use? Which are heart healthy? Why?

4. Your heart needs the right food and exercise. Make up an 8-minute aerobic exercise to do before eating your pizza

2. What are your team's favorite pizza toppings? Which are heart-healthy? Why?

3. A healthy pizza includes items from the four food groups. What are these groups? What pizza ingredients belong in each group?

Fig. 9.3. Pizza puzzler

Handout 9.2   Week 9, Family Activity: Family Fitness Log

Complete with a family member, preferably a parent.

Name_____

Family member_____

	Activity	**Time of day**	**Duration**
Monday	_____	_____	_____
Tuesday	_____	_____	_____
Wednesday	_____	_____	_____
Thursday	_____	_____	_____
Friday	_____	_____	_____
Saturday	_____	_____	_____
Sunday	_____	_____	_____

Instructions

1. Use a different color pen for yourself and for your selected family member.
2. List the activity and in parentheses, indicate the number of minutes (e.g., bicycling 10 mins).
3. Record all activity, including recess, physical education, and sports practice time.
4. Label activity, Morning (M), Afternoon (A), Evening (E).
5. Record the time your log begins and ends.
6. Record the total activity time per week.

Students can rate exercise based on pulse rate and perceived exertion scale (see handout 2.3).

Time: 20 minutes

Please return by_____.

Lesson Elements

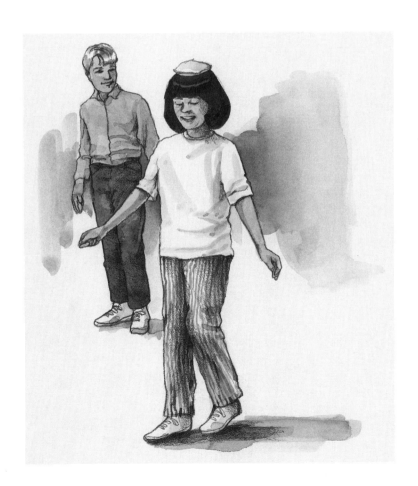

Stretching Routines

Routine 1

For use on the playground (outside) where students cannot lie on the ground (see fig. 10.1).

A. Neck

Keeping shoulders back and spine straight, slowly roll the head to the left shoulder, straighten; then roll toward right shoulder, straighten. Repeat five times. Do not roll head in a fast, circular manner or roll head backward.

B. Back stretch (for shoulder and upper arm)

Lift right arm and reach behind head and down the spine. With left hand, push down on right elbow and hold. Reverse arm positions and repeat.

C. Side bender (sides of body)

Stretch left arm overhead to right. Bend to right at waist, reaching as far to right as possible with the left arm; reach as far as possible to the left with right arm, hold. Repeat on opposite side.

D. Knee pumps (back of legs)

While standing, hold the left leg behind the knee and draw it toward your chest. Hold 10 seconds, switch legs, and repeat three times.

E. Heel and toe raise (calf muscles)

Stand with feet close together, hands on hips. Raise up on toes, then heels. Repeat three times.

F. Hip circles (midsection)

Keeping feet and head still, slowly rotate the hips in a sweeping circular motion to loosen the midsection. Repeat five times and change direction.

Routine 2

For use inside a gym, multipurpose room, or classroom where students can lie on the floor to stretch (see fig. 10.2).

A. Neck

Keeping shoulders back and spine straight, slowly roll the head to the left shoulder, straighten; then roll toward right shoulder, straighten. Repeat five times. Do not roll head in fast, circular manner or roll head backward.

B. Knee to nose touch (legs and stomach)

In an all fours position, lift the knee to touch the nose. Move the leg back so the leg does not lift higher than the hips, and the neck and lower back are not hyperextended.

C. Shin stretcher (shins)

Kneel on both knees, turn to right and press down on right ankle with right hand and hold. Keep hips thrust forward to avoid hyperflexing knees. Do not sit on heels. Repeat on left side.

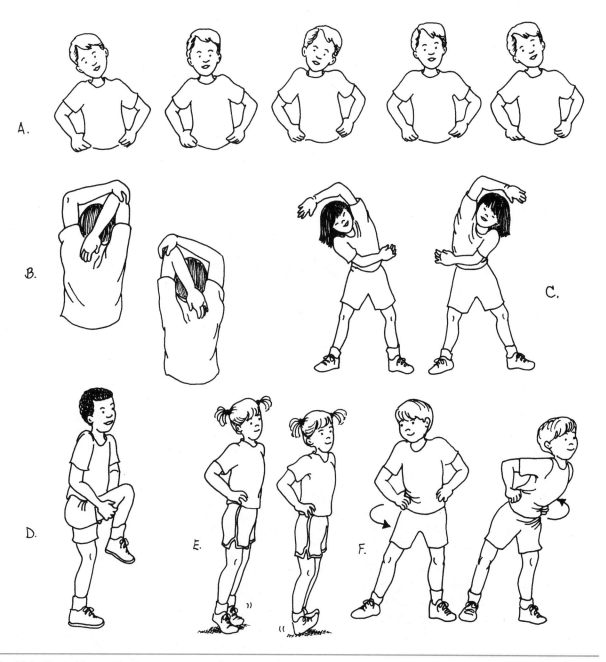

Fig. 10.1. Stretching routine 1

D. Single leg tuck (back of leg and lower back)

Sit on floor with left leg straight. Tuck right foot against left thigh. Lower chest toward left knee. Repeat with right leg.

E. Low-back stretch (low-back muscle)

Lie on back and tuck knees to chest.

Routine 3

For use inside a gym, multipurpose room, or classroom where students can lie on the floor to stretch (see fig. 10.3).

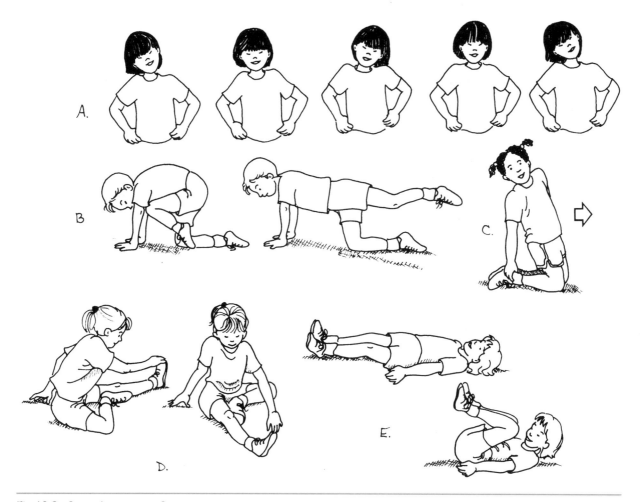

Fig. 10.2. Stretching routine 2

A. Sitting stretch (inside of thighs)

Sit with soles of feet together, place hands on knees or ankles, and lean forearms against knees. Resist while attempting to raise knees.

B. Behind neck grasp (back of arms)

Lift right arm and reach behind head and down the spine. With the left hand, reach behind back and grasp the right hand. Reverse hands.

C. One leg stretcher (lower back and back of legs)

Stand with one foot on a bench, keeping both legs straight. Press down on bench with the heel for several seconds; then relax and bend the trunk forward, trying to touch the head to the knee. Hold for a few seconds. Return to starting position and repeat with opposite leg. As flexibility increases, the arms can pull the chest toward the legs. Do not lock knee.

D. Arm stretcher (arms and chest)

Cross arms and turn palms of hands together. Raise arms overhead behind ears. Extend at the elbows. Reach as high as possible.

E. Trunk twister (midsection and waist)

Sit with right leg extended, left leg bent and crossed over right knee. Place right arm on the left side of the left leg, and push against that leg while turning the trunk as far as possible to the left. Place left hand on floor behind buttocks. Reverse position and repeat on opposite side.

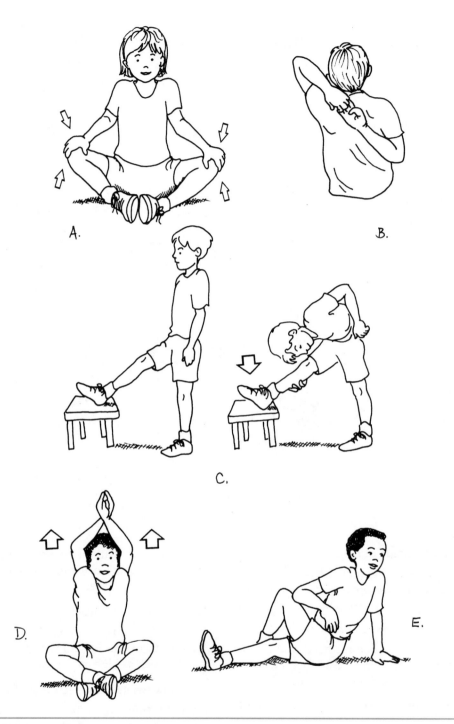

Fig. 10.3. Stretching routine 3

Warm-Up Activities

Select warm-ups that allow easy transition to the main activity of lesson. For example, the first warm-up would be ideal if the main focus of the lesson is jumping rope. The equipment is already available.

Jump rope and stretch

One rope per student. Each student has jump rope and slowly starts jumping. On signal, the student performs a stretch using the jump rope. An example would be to fold the rope in half and hold it overhead while bending from side to side and to the toes.

Ready, draw!

With partners, each player starts with hands behind their backs. On "Draw," the players show either one or two fingers. If the players show different numbers, they do 10 repetitions of an exercise, for example, jumping jacks. If they show the same numbers, they do nothing and "Draw" again.

Line jump

Students stand next to a line on the playground or in the gym. They jump from side to side without touching the line for 30 seconds. How many times did you cross the line? Try again to see if your score improves.

Triangle tag

In groups of four, two students face each other and hold hands. The other two stand on either side of the students holding hands. One person is "it" and chased by the other. The two holding hands act as a shield to the one being chased.

Fifteen-second gusto

After some light running, complete the following:

15 seconds of jumping jacks

15 seconds of sit-ups

15 seconds of line jumps

15 seconds of jogging on the spot bringing knees up high

15 seconds of modified push-ups

Court line tag

Students play on a basketball court, scattering anywhere on lines. All tags are made below the shoulder with Nerf balls. The two taggers, who tag with Nerf balls, start in the center. During game, players must stay on lines. If tagged, a player takes Nerf ball and immediately becomes a new tagger. Original tagger cannot be immediately tagged.

Kanga ball

In groups of three, two partners face each other and roll a ball back and forth. The third child stands between the pair and jumps over the ball, but turns to keep an eye on it. Roll the ball slowly at first. The objective is not to hit the player in the middle, but to make the player jump. Players can kick the ball back and forth or sit with their legs spread and roll the ball. The jumper can ask the others to vary the speed or keep it the same, according to ability. You can use balls of different sizes, and children change roles after 45 seconds.

Cigarette pack

This game is like smoking cigarettes. The more you smoke, the more difficulty you have being active. Designate one area of gym or playground as playing area. Select one person to be the cigarette, who chases others and tags them. The tagged players hook elbows or join hands and continue chasing others. The "cigarette chain" grows and grows. As it does, it has more difficulty moving. Split into two after chain reaches 6 players.

Partner cruise

Begin the activity with the students walking in a scatter formation around the gym. On command, have each student find a partner to face and shake their hand. This person is designated their "Handshake" partner. Again, the students scatter throughout the gym. On command, they must find their Handshake partners and shake hands. They then find a second partner and create a different handshake. The activity continues with students finding different partners and doing a different action with each partner, such as Back to Back, High Five, Sole Shake, and so on. Between partners, the students walk or jog.

Over and under

Students find a partner. One partner makes a bridge on the floor while the other moves over, under, and around the bridge. This continues until you give a signal to switch, which notifies them to change positions. Try different types of bridges and movements.

Weave run

The entire class starts walking counterclockwise in a circle around a designated area (e.g., track, gym, softball diamond). One student is the lead runner and one is the back runner. On signal, the back runner weaves in and out of the runners to the front. Then each runner in turn weaves their way to the front. When each runner has weaved while group is walking, tell students to jog and repeat run.

Leader of the pack

Form groups of four to six students. Designate a leader, and students form a line behind leader. Leader runs and the line follows. Leader determines movement pattern and is allowed to jog, run slowly, skip, hop, run sideways or backward. You can permit other movements after students become familiar with task. Every 30 seconds, change leader.

Partner jog

Students find a partner and stand side by side, ready to run. On the signal "Go," students run slowly side by side with partner in designated area. On the signal "Change," pairs split up and find a new partner. Students greet new partner.

Hexagonal run and jump

Mark out a hexagonal shape with six cones. Students jog around the hexagon. In the middle of each side of the hexagon, students stop and jump into the hexagon, back out again, and continue jogging. Encourage different types of jumps (e.g., one foot, two feet).

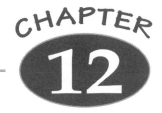

Cool-Down Activities

Select cool-downs that allow an easy transition. For example, if children are already in pairs, Car Mania cool-down may be appropriate.

Rhythm run

Students form pairs and jog side by side around a baseball diamond or basketball court. Instruct them to run so their left and right feet move in rhythm together. When they can do this in pairs, have them progress to groups of four. Encourage students to remind their running partner to use good running techniques. Slowly change from jogging to walking.

Slo-mo skip

Set up four cones in square (40 × 40 yards). Students start by skipping one circuit at a fast rate, and each circuit thereafter slow down a little until they are in slo-mo.

Birthday line

Tell the students that they can no longer talk. The group challenge is to see how effectively the class can arrange themselves in order of birthdays from January 1 at one end to December 31 at the other end. They can use sign language but cannot talk. Have them complete some stretches when they are in line.

Car mania

In pairs, one child puts a hula hoop around the waist of the other child. The first child steers the other around the playground or gym. Children can use gears and gradually slow down.

Progressive relaxation

Students tense different muscle groups for 10 seconds and then relax. Use music that is relaxing. Students lie on back with legs slightly apart and arms at sides. Think of something pleasant. Press head against mat and relax. Frown and move scalp upward. Squeeze shoulder blades together and relax. Make fists with hands and relax. Tighten tummy muscles and relax. Press legs to floor and relax. Point toes and relax.

Around the group

Arrange students in two lines, side by side. Lines stay side by side and jog. On a signal, the last pair in line runs to the front of the line. Once this pair reaches the front of the line, the next pair runs from the back. This continues until all pairs have run from back. Then slow down to a walk.

Grid jog

Mark out four squares 10 × 10 yards with cones. Students have to jog to each square in turn and complete one repetition of their favorite exercise. After jogging to each square, students then walk to each square in turn and complete one repetition of their exercise.

Figure 8

Place two cones 30 yards apart. Students move single file around the cones in a figure 8 pattern. Call out the movements starting with jogging, skipping, or galloping, gradually reducing to a walk.

Jog and stretch

Set up four stretching stations around playing area. Divide class into four groups. After completing 30 seconds at a stretching station, a group jogs two laps around area and moves to next station.

Run and split

The class jogs single file down the middle of the playing area. At the end of the area, they split, one person goes to the left, the next to the right, and so on. Runners run around the perimeter of the square. When they return to the starting point, they run side by side down the middle and go to their same direction at the end of the area. Finish by walking through the pattern.

Exercises

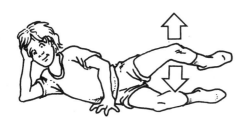

Sit-ups. Lie on back with knees bent (12–18 inch gap between feet and buttocks) and arms across chest. Lift upper body toward knees until arms touch thighs and lower until midback touches floor.

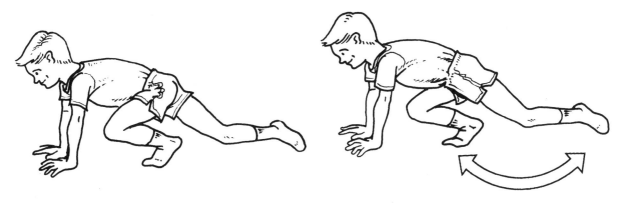

Mountain climbers. In front support position, bring the right knee up under chest and extend the left leg backward. Quickly switch leg positions, keeping a rhythmic movement pattern.

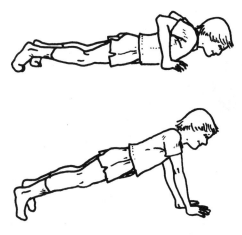

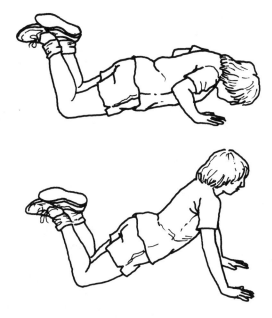

Push-ups. Lie on stomach with chest touching floor and feet together. Hands are under the shoulders. Push and raise body by extending arms. Raise body in straight line, not allowing back to sway. Lower body until chin touches ground.

Modified push-ups. Do as regular push-ups, only push up from knees, not feet.

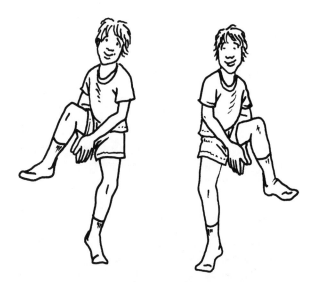

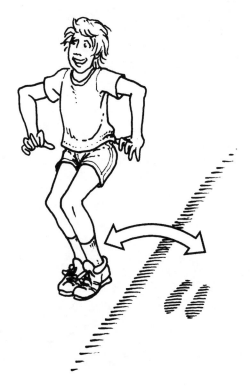

Clappers. Hop on left foot, kick the right leg up, and clap your hands under the right leg. Hop on the right foot, kick the left leg up, and clap your hands under it. Land on the ball of the foot each time.

Skier. With both feet together, jump from side to side over a line or jump rope.

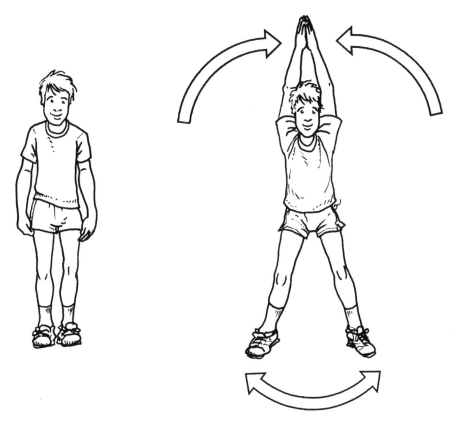

Jumping jacks.   Stand with arms by sides. Simultaneously raise arms above head and move legs shoulder-width apart. Then bring arms to sides and feet together.

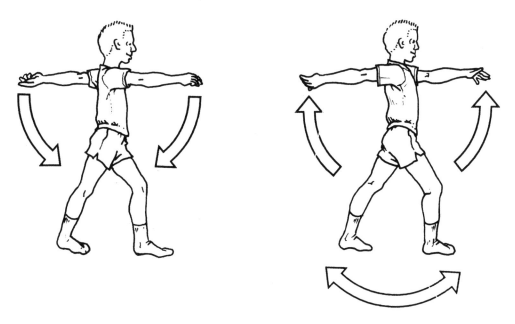

Cross-country skier.   Stand with one foot in front and one foot behind body. The opposite arm is also in front of the body. Jump and change positions of feet and arms.

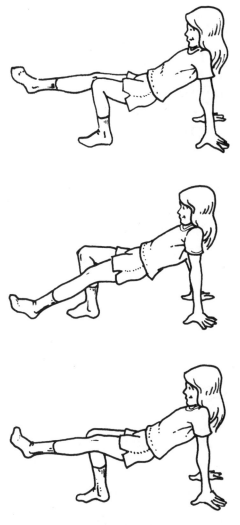

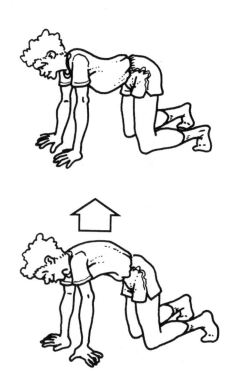

Bridge back. On hands and knees in a crawling position, contract abdominal muscles and arch back as high as possible. Return to starting position.

Crab legs. Support weight on hands and feet. Alternatively kick legs out away from body. Each kick counts as one repetition.

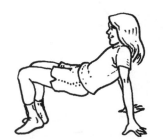 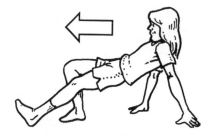 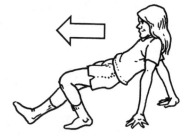

Crab walker. From sitting position, push body off the ground and support weight on hands and feet. Move body forward three steps and backward three steps.

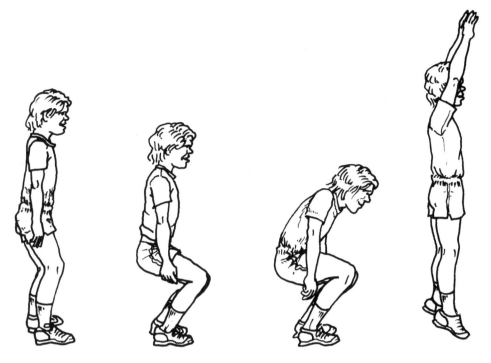

Jack-in-the-box.   Squat down low and pretend you are hiding in a box. Spring up reaching as high as you can. Return to starting position.

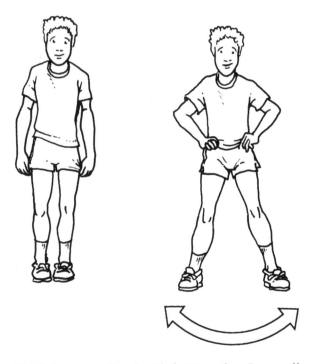

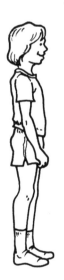 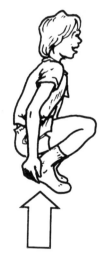

Heel touches.   Stand in an upright position with feet shoulder-width apart and arms fully extended at the sides. Jump vertically and touch the heels with the hands as the knees move to the chest.

Stride jumps.   Stand with feet together. Jump off ground so feet are spread three feet apart. Return to starting position.

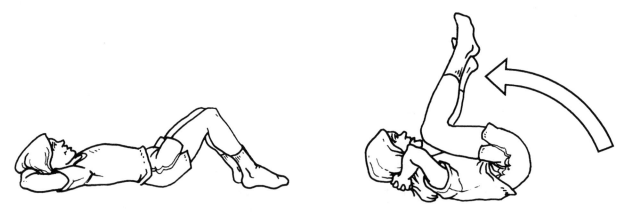

Reverse sit-ups.   Lie on back with legs together and knees bent. Bend at the waist and bring knees to chest. Lower legs to starting position.

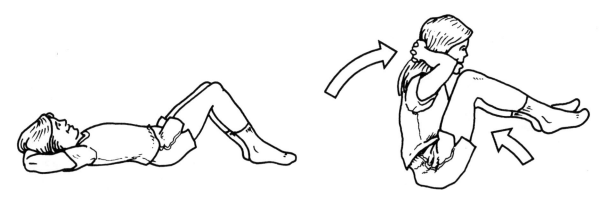

Crunches.   Lie on back with legs together and legs and knees bent, forming a 90-degree angle. Hands are behind head. Bring knees and elbows together, directly over waist area. Return to starting position.

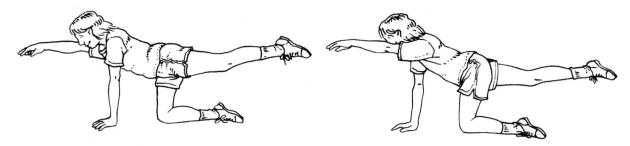

Cross body lift.   Assume an all fours position with your hands on the floor directly under your shoulders. In this position, raise one arm and the opposite leg simultaneously until they are slightly higher than your back. Then lower both simultaneously. Repeat this action with the opposite arm and leg in alternating fashion.

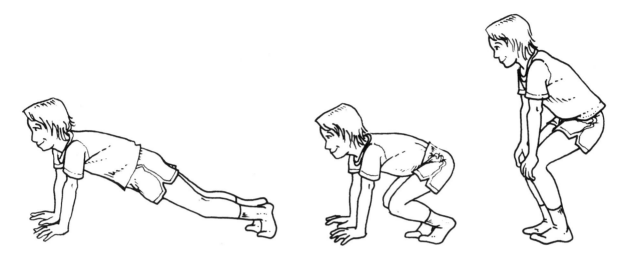

Squat thrusts.   In push-up position quickly move legs toward hands and jump high into the air.

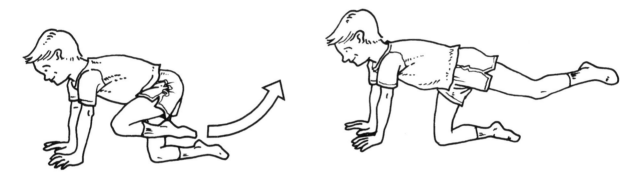

Leg extensions.   On all fours with legs square and right knee bent, raise right leg to side. Extend your leg forward and backward, parallel to the floor, then lower to the ground. Move legs only and keep upper body still. Change legs.

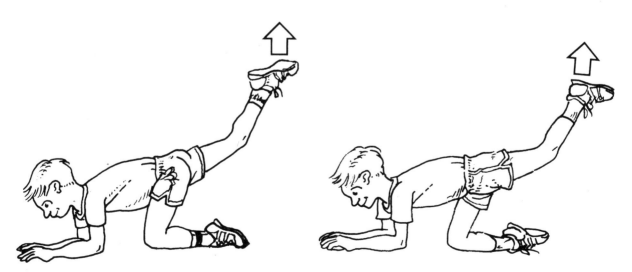

Skyscrapers.   Kneel on all fours. Lower weight to forearms and tighten abdominal muscles. Raise bent leg behind and push it to the ceiling. Flex and point the foot.

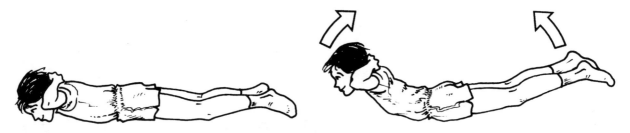

Chest raises.   Lie on stomach with feet together and hands clasped behind head. Raise head and chest away from ground and slowly lower to starting position.

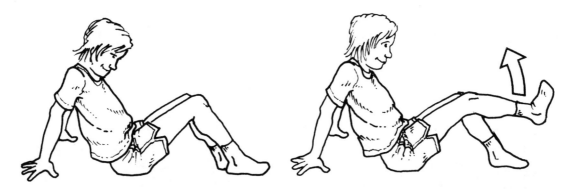

Thigh lifts.   Begin in the half-hook, half-long sit position. Raise and lower the extended leg. Change leg and raise.

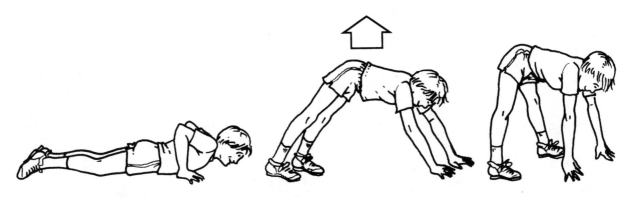

Inchworm.   Lie on stomach. Keep hands still and take small steps forward toward your hands. Then move feet back away from hands to the lying position.

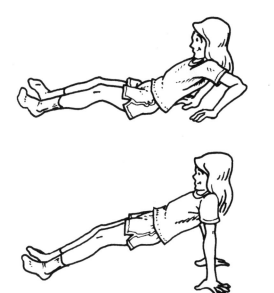

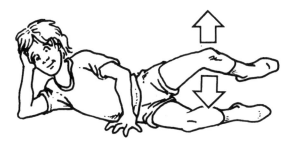

Side leg raises.   Lie on your right side with your head resting on your right hand and your left hand flat on the mat in front of you for support. Raise your upper leg. Repeat, changing sides.

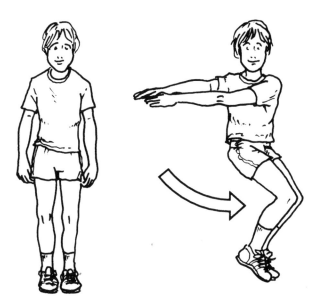

Reverse push-ups.   In back support position, bend elbows to slowly lower body to the floor. Straighten elbows to raise body away from floor.

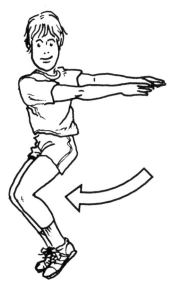

Jump twisters.   Stand with feet together, knees slightly bent. Thrust both arms to right while moving legs (from waist) to the left. Reverse action with arms moving to the left and legs to the right.

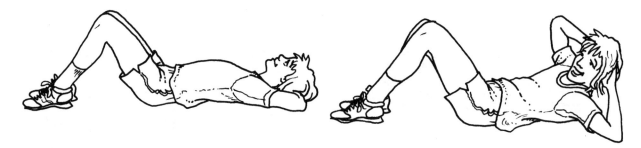

Obliques. Lie on back with knees bent, feet on floor with hands held lightly behind head. Lift shoulder and upper torso off the floor twisting one elbow toward opposite knee. Do not pull head and neck with hands. Return to starting position and repeat on other side. Press spine to floor so hips do not roll.

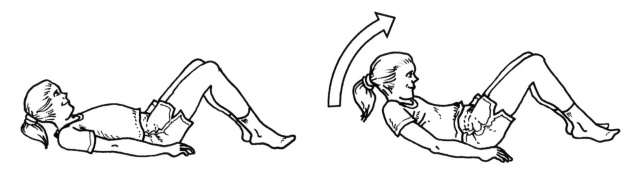

Curl-ups. Lie on back with knees at a 90-degree angle and arms extended by side. Lift head until upper back is raised from floor and the chin touches the chest. Return to floor.

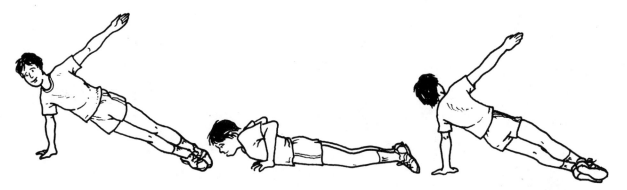

Side standers. Lie on stomach with chest touching floor. Raise body in push-up fashion and rotate body so you support weight on right hand and foot. Return to starting position and support weight on left hand and foot.

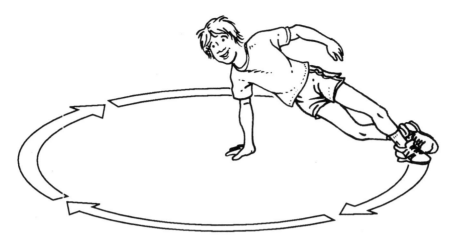

Coffee grinder.   Pivot on a supporting hand. Work feet around hand making a complete circle while keeping the body straight.

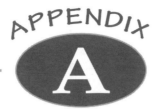

APPENDIX

A

Physical Fitness Testing

Physical fitness testing has traditionally been a part of physical education. We believe this should continue, but with the following concepts clearly in mind:

- Teach children to test themselves. Children who learn to test themselves will know their current fitness levels and develop skills to use in later life.
- Self-evaluation, rather than comparison to others is important. Heredity, maturity, and age have much to do with fitness performance. Use test results to help students plan personal fitness programs.
- Explain why fitness testing is important. Reaching acceptable health fitness standards provided by programs, helping children identify their own strengths and weaknesses, and allowing children to monitor their improvement are all good reasons for physical fitness testing.
- If you are going to use awards, clearly explain the procedure for receiving awards. Use an incentive program that rewards participation and effort.

The following physical fitness test programs are available:

Physical Best
American Alliance for Health, Physical Education, Recreation and Dance
1900 Association Drive
Reston, VA 22091.

President's Challenge
President's Council on Physical Fitness and Sports
450 Fifth Street NW, Room 7103
Washington, DC 20001.

Physical Fitness Program
Amateur Athletic Union
Poplars Building
Bloomington, IN 47405.

Fitnessgram
Institute for Aerobic Fitness Research
12330 Preston Road
Dallas, TX 74230
1-800-635-7050.

Name: _____

Post Test

Directions: Circle or underline the best response.

1. **As a result of jogging, swimming, or jumping rope for an extended period of at least three times per week, the heart:**

   a. pumps more blood with each beat

   b. may beat slower while resting

   c. may increase in size and strength

   d. all of the above

2. **The pulse indicates:**

   a. how many blood cells are in the body

   b. how fast a person is breathing

   c. how fast a person's heart is beating

   d. all of the above

3. **To gain aerobic fitness benefits, a person must exercise for at least _____ minutes in a workout.**

   a. 5

   b. 10

   c. 20

   d. 30

4. **Cardiovascular exercise involves the:**

   a. heart

   b. lungs

   c. blood vessels

   d. all of the above

5. **The recommended way to loose fat or to keep from becoming fat is to:**

   a. exercise frequently and eat a balanced diet

   b. eat only once a day

   c. stop eating foods that have added sugar in them

   d. go on a diet

6. **Flexibility is the ability to:**

   a. run fast

   b. run for long distances

   c. lift heavy weights

   d. bend and stretch easily

7. **People exercise to:**

   a. have fun

   b. control their weight and look better

   c. keep healthy

   d. all of the above

8. **To become physically fit, a person needs to:**

   a. eat nutritionally sound meals

   b. exercise frequently

   c. get sufficient sleep

   d. all of the above

9. **A child or adult with good cardiovascular fitness, would have a resting heart rate of:**

   a. lower than 70 beats per minute

   b. 70 to 75 beats per minute

   c. 75 to 80 beats per minute

   d. at least 80 beats per minute

10. **Weak abdominal muscles could result in:**

    a. lower back pain

    b. protruding abdomen

    c. poor posture

    d. all of the above

11. **It is generally accepted that to be fit and healthy, a person needs to do aerobic exercise for 20 minutes a minimum of:**

    a. one day per week

    b. two days per week

    c. three days per week

    d. seven days per week

12. **A cool down is important after vigorous exercise because:**

    a. the pulse rate can return to normal slowly

    b. it helps remove lactic acid from the muscular system

    c. it helps eliminate blood pooling in the legs

    d. all of the above

13. **What would be the safest way to loose weight:**

    a. drink eight glasses of water each day and eat only fruits and vegetables

    b. reduce caloric intake by skipping lunch

    c. "fast" for three days and then begin exercising

    d. reduce caloric intake and increase physical activity

14. **Your best friend says a candy bar is the best snack for energy so he eats at least one a day. You say**

    a. this is true because candy bars have a lot of sugar.

    b. candy bars have a lot of sugar, which eats up your energy.

    c. other snacks provide energy and greater amounts of other nutrients at the same time.

    d. candy bars provide calories, not energy.

15. **Approximately how much salt (sodium) does the body need per day?**

    a. one teaspoon salt (2,500 milligrams sodium)

    b. one half teaspoon salt (1,250 milligrams sodium)

    c. one third teaspoon salt (835 milligrams sodium)

16. **Which of the following commonly eaten foods are high in salt (sodium)?**

    a. Cheerios

    b. cottage cheese

    c. meat

    d. apple

17. **Which of the following should you avoid to lower the total intake of fat in the diet?**

    a. roasting

    b. broiling

    c. frying

    d. barbequing

18. **Which of the following protein sources does not contain cholesterol?**

    a. roast beef

    b. tuna fish

    c. rice

    d. cheese

19. **Which of the following will help reduce the fat content of the diet?**

    a. substitute whole-milk cheese instead of meat

    b. substitute meat instead of fish and poultry

    c. substitute skim milk instead of whole milk

    d. all of the above

20. **The ingredients on a package label are**

    a. in alphabetical order.

    b in descending order by weight.

    c. with nutrients first, additives second, and preservatives last.

    d. at random.

Name: _____

Open-Ended Assessment

1. **Return to sender**

   Ask students to write letters to their "self" from their "body." Suggest an opening line for students, such as the following:

   Hello, this is your body. I will let you know how you have been looking after me.

   Students can also write a response letter from the "self" to the "body" in which they identify lifestyle modifications for improving health. You can use letters to develop discussion around the importance of lifestyle changes. This approach helps personalize the health-fitness concept. Letters can also include specific goals for students.

2. **Health hints**

   Ask students to design their own Healthy Heart Tip Sheet. Tell them to prepare a sheet for their family. The tips should be presented along with graphics and work that students can design.

3. **From the store to the stage**

   Work with a partner to prepare a skit about heart-healthy eating. Include selection, preparation, and consumption of food. Perform skit for classmates.

4. **Fit thinking**

   Inside the "Fit Thinking" outline (see fig. A.1), record the thoughts of someone who is concerned about their personal health. Draw symbols or write words or phrases that represent ideas about developing an exercise program and improving eating habits.

5. **Excuses! Excuses!**

   Students identify exercises and activities in which they commonly participate. Explain why people select different activities or exercises for many reasons, including the following:

   1. For enjoyment
   2. To feel better
   3. To fit easily into everyday routine
   4. To do near school, home, or work
   5. To do no matter what weather or season
   6. To develop physical fitness

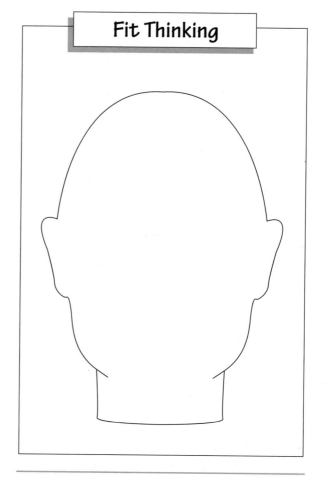

Fig. A.1. Fit thinking

On a sheet of paper tell students to list all the activities that are part of a typical day (e.g., sleeping, washing, personal hygiene, watching TV, sitting in school). Have the children estimate the number of hours and minutes involved in each activity. Ask the students to share their use of time with the class. Avoid making value statements. Instead, emphasize preferable activities. Especially encourage those that include physical activity.

When it comes to exercising, too many people are long on excuses and short on "just doing it," as a recent sneaker commercial points out. Have students write on slips of paper possible excuses for avoiding exercise. Put all slips in a box, and have each child select one.

Have students write a persuasive letter about the value of exercise and the inadequacy of the excuse. They should also include suggestions for eliminating the excuse. For example, for the excuse, "I planned to go for a bike ride, but it started to rain," someone might suggest alternative indoor activities, such as riding a stationary bike or jumping rope for 10 minutes. Post letters on a "Just Do It!" bulletin board, or create cartoon bubbles in which one cartoon is an excuse and the other cartoon is an alternative.

6. **Just stay with it!**

Analyze the data from the weekly exercise plans from lesson 41. Calculate total minutes per day in activities. Review time of day of exercise. Is there a specific pattern? Were students more active in the morning, afternoon, or evening? Which activities were aerobic? Did they include a warm-up and cool-down? Do you think the results would be the same summer and winter? Does weather affect your choice of activity? Students can bar graph number of minutes per day spent exercising.

7. **Fitness clubs**

Continue the theme started in lesson 43 on Fitness Clubs. Students can select various activities around a central theme (e.g., soccer, jump rope, basketball, running, walking, or other activities). Students design a cardiovascular workout using skills with other club members. Students plan a complete workout lesson including warm-up, workout, and cool-down. Students can also prepare a list of materials.

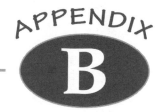
Parent Letter

You may use this sample letter as a guide for informing parents of the program and soliciting their involvement, or you may want to develop your own format. The goal for the program is to improve attitudes toward fitness in both students and parents, and to increase communication between the home and school.

Dear Parents:

Your child will be participating in a new physical fitness program soon. The name of the program is Health-Related Fitness. It will begin on (date) and run approximately _____ weeks.

In this program, we will explore a variety of topics related to health, physical fitness, and nutrition. We will emphasize establishing healthy habits that will last a lifetime. Students will learn how to assess their individual fitness level based on the knowledge they gain in this program and will be able to design their personal fitness program. They will learn how to maintain a healthy level of physical fitness. Also, they will learn about heart-healthy nutrition and how to improve their eating habits.

Your child will be involved in a wide range of fitness and nutrition activities. The weekly schedule is three days of physical activity and two days of classroom instruction. Students will be expected to perform only at their own level. Our goal is to help each student strive for and recognize individual gains in his or her fitness level.

If you have questions or would like further information about this program, please contact me by phone or letter. You will be receiving information about Family Fitness activities. We hope you will be able to participate and enjoy the fun with your children. We hope you can give support and encouragement to your child for continued improvement in health and fitness.

Please call me if you have any questions.

Sincerely,

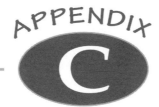

APPENDIX C

Additional Resources

Bennett, J.P., and A. Kamiya. 1986. *Fitness and fun for everyone.* Durham, NC: Great Activities.

Cames, C. 1983. *Awesome elementary school physical education activities.* Carmichael, CA: Education.

Corbin, C.B., and R.P. Pangrazi. 1990. *Teaching strategies for improving youth fitness.* Dallas: Institute for Aerobics Research.

Foster, E.R., K. Hartinger, and K.A. Smith. 1992. *Fitness fun.* Champaign, IL: Human Kinetics.

Hopper, C. 1988. *The sports confident child.* New York: Pantheon Books.

Landy, J.M., and M.L. Landy. 1992. *Ready-to-use P.E. activities for grades K-2.* West Nyack, NY: Parker.

Pangrazi, R.P., and V.P. Dauer. 1992. *Dynamic physical education for elementary school children.* New York: Macmillan.

Petray, C.K., and S.L. Blazer. 1987. *Health-related physical fitness.* Edina, MN: Burgess.

Stillwell, J.L., and J.R. Stockard. 1988. *More fitness activities for children.* Durham, NC: Great Activities.

Index

About the Authors

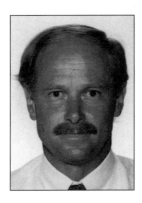

Chris Hopper, PhD, is department chair and professor of physical education at Humboldt State University in Arcata, California.

Hopper brings a variety of experiences in physical education to his writing. Since 1976 he has taught physical education at the elementary through college level. He also has consulted with a variety of organizations, including the United States Department of Education, the Boys Clubs of America, and the American Sport Education Program. Throughout his career he has coached both youth and collegiate soccer, serving as head coach of men's soccer at Humboldt State University.

In 1982 Hopper earned his PhD in physical education from the University of Oregon. Much of his research has focused on improving children's physical fitness and nutrition. He has published numerous articles in the *Journal of Physical Education, Recreation and Dance; Scholastic Coach; Adapted Physical Activity Quarterly;* and the *Research Quarterly for Exercise and Sport.* He is coauthor of *Coaching Soccer Effectively* and author of *The Sports-Confident Child.*

Hopper is a member of the American Alliance for Health, Physical Education, Recreation and Dance, the National Consortium on Physical Education and Recreation for Individuals With Disabilities; and the American Council on Rural Special Education.

Hopper, who lives in Ferndale, California, with his wife, Renee, and their three children, enjoys soccer, golf, and waterskiing.

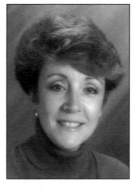

Kathy D. Munoz, EdD, is assistant professor in the Department of Health and Physical Education at Humboldt State University.

Munoz has a master's in food and nutrition from Oregon State University and an EdD in education and curriculum design from the University of Southern California. As a registered dietitian and home economics teacher, she has taught nutrition to a wide variety of ages and backgrounds, including secondary, community college, and university students. She also worked with students, athletes, and community members as a counselor at the Eating Disorder Clinic in Humboldt.

In 1989 Munoz won the Meritorious Performance and Professional Promise Award from Humboldt State for teaching nutrition. She is advisor to the Youth Education Services (YES) Nutrition for Kids program, a role she filled also for the Student Home Economics Association.

A member of the American Dietetic Association, American College of Nutrition, and the Society for Nutrition Education, Munoz lives in Fortuna, California, with her husband, Richard, and their three children. She pursues outdoor sports, reading, and traveling in her spare time.

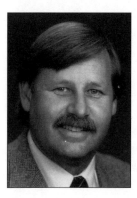

Bruce Fisher has received several honors for teaching excellence, including 1991 California Teacher of the Year, 1991 Professional Best Award, and the ABC-TV Favorite Teacher Award. A classroom teacher since 1975, he has created meaningful activities and lessons to teach fitness and nutrition to students at all grade levels.

As a member of the California State Department of Education's Health and Physical Education committee since 1991, Fisher helped design and develop the health and physical education frameworks for California. He has served on educational and curriculum development committees throughout his career, including the Family Wellness Project, and he also has presented at education conferences across the country.

In 1991 Fisher wrote the feature article for *Learning Magazine* on health and nutrition. Now with the Jet Propulsion Lab, Johns Hopkins University, and San Diego State University, he is writing the curriculum for NASA's KidSat/ Project YES.

Fisher lives in Fieldbrook, California, with his wife, Mindi, and their daughter, Jenny. His hobbies include aviation, aerospace, astronomy, and photography.

Integrate health and fitness lessons into your curriculum with these ready-to-use activities

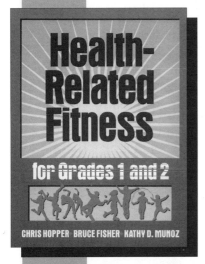

1996 • Paper • 128 pp
Item BHOP0498
ISBN 0-87322-498-1
$16.00 ($23.95 Canadian)

1996 • Paper • 136 pp
Item BHOP0499
ISBN 0-87322-499-X
$16.00 ($23.95 Canadian)

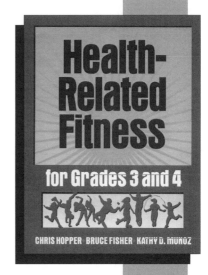

1996 • Paper • Approx 160 pp
Item BHOP0480
ISBN 0-88011-480-0
$18.00 ($26.95 Canadian)

Each *Health-Related Fitness* book provides 45 grade-appropriate, cross-curricular lessons and activities in physical fitness and nutrition. The classroom-tested programs in each book provide nine weeks of plans for five 30-minute, ready-to-use lessons.

This unique, hands-on curriculum includes homework assignments with family activities, cooperative learning experiences, cross-curricular activities to stimulate critical thinking skills, reproducible handouts, easy-to-understand adaptable scripts, activities based on state and national health standards, and lessons that require either no equipment or simple materials readily available.

Part I of each book outlines lessons on cardiovascular fitness, strength, endurance, flexibility, and nutrition to help you prepare students for a healthy lifestyle. **Part II** describes the different kinds of elements you should teach in each lesson, including stretches, warm-ups, cool-downs, and exercises.

Special Package Price

All 3 *Health-Related Fitness* books • Item BHOP0668 • ISBN 0-88011-668-4
$43.00 ($64.50 Canadian)

Human Kinetics
The Information Leader in Physical Activity
http://www.humankinetics.com/

2335

Prices are subject to change.

To place your order, U.S. customers **call TOLL FREE 1-800-747-4457**.
Customers outside the U.S. place your order using the appropriate
telephone number/address shown in the front of this book.